# KETO DIET LUNCH ON THE GO

Quick & Easy Ketogenic Recipes You Can Prepare At Home For Packing Lunch On The Go

Ted Duncan

# Contents

**What is a ketogenic diet?** ................................................................. 7

**Benefits Of Ketosis** ........................................................................... 9

**Getting Started With Ketogenic Diet** ........................................ 10

**Additional Points of Interest** ..................................................... 12

**Foods Recommended On Ketogenic Diet** ............................... 13

**Foods To Avoid On Ketogenic Diet** .......................................... 15

**Lunch Recipes** ................................................................................ 16

    Keto Pistachio Tomato Avocado Toast ................................................ 16

    Keto Eggplant Burger .............................................................................. 19

    Loaded Cauliflower Bake ........................................................................ 22

    Low Carb Keto Meatloaf ......................................................................... 25

    Curry Chicken Lettuce Wraps ................................................................ 28

    Low Carb High Fat Chicken Nuggets ..................................................... 31

    Chicken Vegetable Skillet ....................................................................... 34

    Keto Ham Spinach Mini Quiche ............................................................ 37

    Peach Pan Fried Scallops Salad Recipe ................................................. 39

    Chicken Teriyaki ...................................................................................... 41

    Asian Chicken and Cabbage Salad ........................................................ 44

    Chicken Taco Salad ................................................................................. 48

    Smoked Salmon Keto Wrap ................................................................... 51

    Garlicky Keto Greens .............................................................................. 53

Keto Fish Sticks .................................................................................. 56

Smoky Tuna Pickle Boats .................................................................. 59

Keto Corn Dog Muffins ...................................................................... 61

Slow Cooker Garlic Chipotle Lime Chicken ..................................... 63

Fresh Sriracha Broccoli Salad ........................................................... 66

Keto Chicken Enchilada Bow ............................................................ 68

Keto Broccoli Beef Recipe ................................................................. 71

Garlic Roasted Shrimp with Zucchini Pasta .................................... 73

Chocolate Almond Keto Fat Bomb ................................................... 75

Keto Macaroon Fat Bombs ............................................................... 77

Quick 3-Ingredients Peanut Butter Fudge ...................................... 79

Low Carb Almond Flour Waffles ...................................................... 81

Keto Cream Cheese Truffles ............................................................. 83

Avocado Egg Salad ............................................................................ 85

Basil Scramble .................................................................................... 88

Pomegranate Curry Chicken ............................................................ 90

Blackened Steak Salad ...................................................................... 92

Butter Scallops ................................................................................... 95

Salmon Salad ..................................................................................... 98

Tomato and Basil Chicken .............................................................. 100

Tuna and Tomato Burgers ............................................................. 103

Banana Nut Porridge ...................................................................... 106

Coconut Chicken Fingers ................................................................ 108

Gluten-Free Egg Roll In Bowl ......................................................... 111

Quick and Easy Lunch Scramble ................................................... 113

Good Noon Chicken Burrito Bowls ................................................................ 116

Pizza Frittata ........................................................................................................ 118

Egg Muffin Recipe ............................................................................................. 121

Egg Casseroles .................................................................................................... 124

Grilled Fish Fillet ................................................................................................ 126

Cilantro Lime Shrimp with Zucchini Noodles ........................... 129

Sauted Chicken Mushroom Omlette ............................................. 132

Baked Eggs .......................................................................................................... 135

Chicken Thighs with Shallots And Spinach ................................ 137

Spinach and Cheddar Microwave Quiche .................................. 140

Chicken Breasts with Shaved Brussels Sprouts ...................... 143

© Copyright 2018 by Ted Duncan - All rights reserved.

The follow eBook is reproduced below with the goal of providing information that is as accurate and reliable as possible. Regardless, purchasing this eBook can be seen as consent to the fact that both the publisher and the author of this book are in no way experts on the topics discussed within and that any recommendations or suggestions that are made herein are for entertainment purposes only. Professionals should be consulted as needed prior to undertaking any of the action endorsed herein.

This declaration is deemed fair and valid by both the American Bar Association and the Committee of Publishers Association and is legally binding throughout the United States.

Furthermore, the transmission, duplication or reproduction of any of the following work including specific information will be considered an illegal act irrespective of if it is done electronically or in print. This extends to creating a secondary or tertiary copy of the work or a recorded copy and is only allowed with express written consent from the Publisher. All additional right reserved.

The information in the following pages is broadly considered to be a truthful and accurate account of facts and as such any inattention, use or misuse of the information in question by the reader will render any resulting actions solely under their purview. There are no scenarios in which the publisher or the original author of this work can be in any fashion deemed liable for any hardship or damages that may befall them after undertaking information described herein.

Additionally, the information in the following pages is intended only for informational purposes and should thus be thought of as universal. As befitting its nature, it is presented without assurance regarding its prolonged validity or interim quality. Trademarks that are mentioned are done without written consent and can in no way be considered an endorsement from the trademark holder.

**If you enjoy such content, click below to subscribe where we will send out self-improvement, non-fiction books, tips & information for you to read for FREE!**

**Do leave a good review as well if you found the content useful!**

**Click here -> [http://eepurl.com/c5bzdX](http://eepurl.com/c5bzdX)**

# WHAT IS A KETOGENIC DIET?

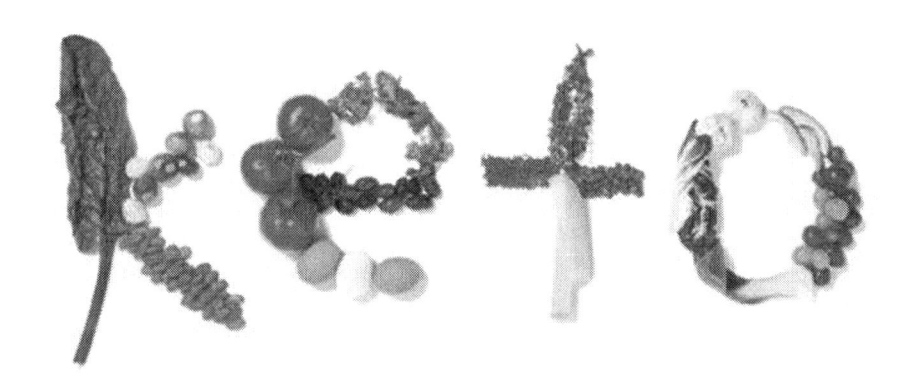

You've probably heard about the *'ketogenic diet'* that's so popular among health-enthusiasts nowadays, and with good reason: this low carb, high fat diet offers complete nourishment with whole foods, making sure that your body burns fat for fuel. In fact, this is the best way to be, as it works wonders to make fat loss mostly effortless! But from where does the word *"ketogenic"* come into the picture?

Well, the word ketogenic is derived from *"ketosis"*, which is essentially that state of your body when it breaks down fat molecules into ketones in order to provide energy. Therefore, one could achieve this state by decreasing the carbohydrate intake and increasing the fat intake.

The "normal" state of the body's metabolism is termed as "glycolysis", in which carbs are burnt for fuel or energy. The bottom is when your body is in carb-burning mode, it will utilize the available carbs to produce energy before it moves to the stored fat. In ketosis, however, your body is programmed to burn fat, which is great news for someone who's trying to get slim and trim.

## BENEFITS OF KETOSIS

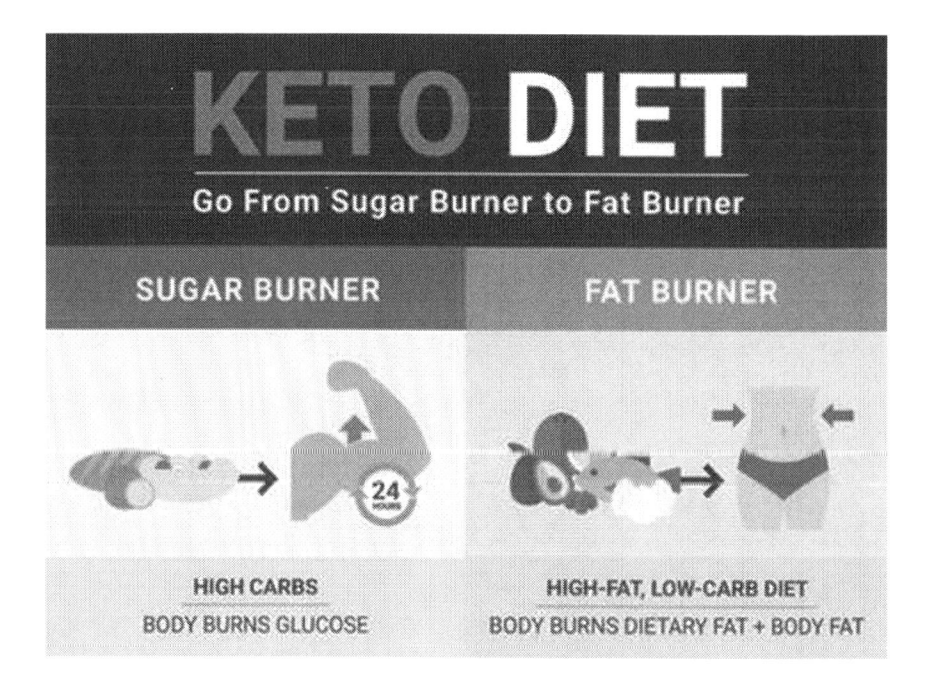

By cutting short the supply of carbs, one can reduce insulin resistance significantly, working as the first line of defense against type-2 diabetes. What's more? When combined with proper exercise, low carb diets could be very effective in alleviating the symptoms and progression of cancer.

Furthermore, ketosis itself is appetite-suppressing, implying that your hunger will check itself naturally, increasing your caloric deficit and making it easier for you to lose fat even faster.

# GETTING STARTED WITH KETOGENIC DIET

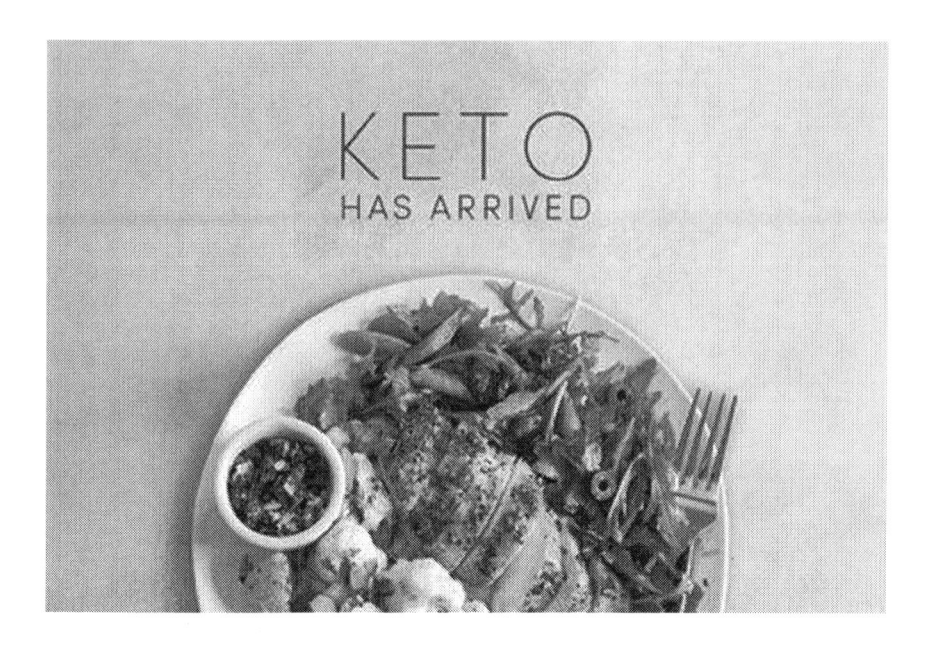

While ketosis may take some time to get in the groove, one requires maintaining at least two weeks of low carb eating for the initial adaptation. Meanwhile, you may experience stints of sluggishness, headaches, fatigue, and some gastrointestinal issues as you become accustomed, often referred to as *"keto flu"*. Don't worry; proper intake of electrolyte will rectify a majority of these issues.

In addition, you must not worry about the "diet" aspect of this ketogenic diet plan – that is **the caloric restriction.** Weight loss will eventually pave its way as your body adapts to the diet and starts to regulate appetite. Moreover, you are strongly recommended to not restrict calories during the initial two weeks as body takes its time to lessen its addiction to sugar and processed food.

The following meal plan is mater-crafted to make sure that you intake balanced yet healthy meals that provide the body with the required amount of fiber, protein and satiation. What sets the ketogenic diet apart from others is the fact that it facilitates muscle loss, whereas other carb-based diets don't. **While the weight-loss in calorie-restricted, high-carb diet will come both from fats and the muscles, keto provides you with the luxury to burn fat without sacrificing muscle.** This is termed as *"body recomposition"* and it gives you a much better physique after weight loss.

## ADDITIONAL POINTS OF INTEREST

The low-carb keto diet often leads to a significant water-loss during the first few phases. Don't worry; this is just because your carbs are being converted into glycogen that is stored in water within the muscles and liver. As you lessen the stored glycogen, your body also flushes this water out. This is the secret to the initial weight loss in first few weeks of ketosis.

While you experience rapid fat loss in the beginning by dropping a significant amount of water, this is a great boost as it results in both weight loss and less bloating, offering a better fitting of clothes to you.

# FOODS RECOMMENDED ON KETOGENIC DIET

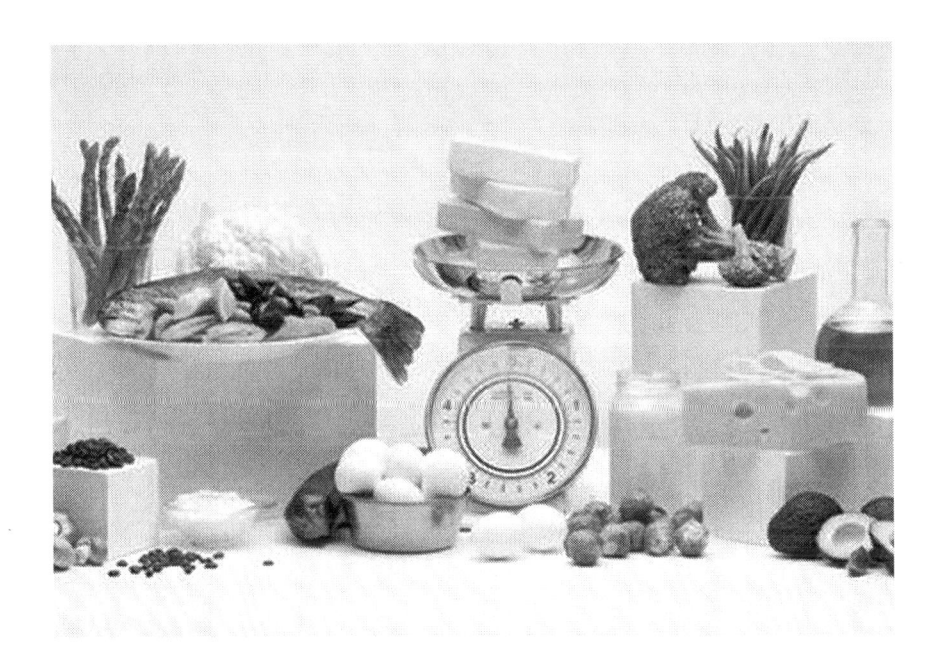

Following a ketogenic diet isn't the easiest thing in the world, especially when you're not sure which foods are recommended to eat. We've deliberately master-crafted a list of ketogenic diet food to help you make better decision what they should eat and shop while following their keto-voyage:

1. **Fats & Oils.** Try to stick to your fat from natural sources such as meat and nuts. Supplement with monounsaturated and saturated fats like coconut oil, butter, and olive oil etc.

2. **Protein.** Try to stick with pasture-raised, organic, and grass-fed meat if possible. A majority of the meets do not boast an added sugar, and so they can be taken in

moderate amount. **Remember:** Consuming a lot of protein on a low-carb diet is not recommended.

3. **Vegetables.** While it doesn't matter if the vegetable is frozen or fresh, what matters more is they are grown above the ground vegetables, and are green in color.

4. **Dairy.** Make sure you buy full-fat dairy items. ***Pro Tip:*** Harder cheeses generally have fewer carbs.

5. **Seeds and Nuts:** In moderation, seeds and nuts could be utilized to create some fantastic textures. You can use fattier nuts like almonds and macadamias.

6. **Beverages.** Keep it simple, sticking to water. If needed, you can flavor it with lemon juice or stevia-based flavorings.

***NOTE***: All of the above foods strictly stick to 5% carb allowance that we have on keto.

# FOODS TO AVOID ON KETOGENIC DIET

1. **Grains:** Includes oats, wheat, barley, corn and rye.

2. **Artificial Sweeteners**: Splenda, Sucralose, Saccharin, etc.

3. **Processed Foods:** If they contain carrageenan, then it is not recommended to eat it.

4. **"Low-fat" products:** Drinks, gluten diet soda, Atkins products, diet soda etc.

# LUNCH RECIPES

## Lunch Recipe 1

## KETO PISTACHIO TOMATO AVOCADO TOAST

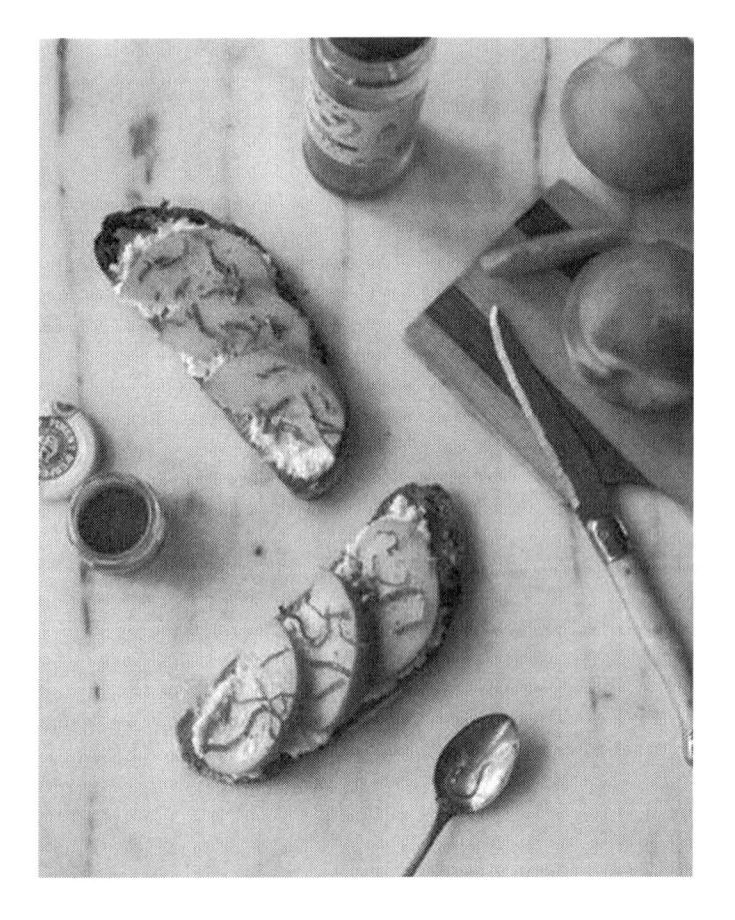

Nutritional value 376 cal
Protein 5 g
Fat 38 g

Carbohydrates 11 g

*An easy to prepare, healthy to eat, and amazingly addicting avocado toast is simply a perfect lunch idea if you were ever to throw a treat to a crowd! This recipe is perfectly Soy-free, Mayo-free, Whole 30 friendly and perfectly keto.*

Serves: 1
Preparation time: 10 minutes
Cooking time: 5 minutes

## Ingredients

1 slice of Keto bread (toasted)
½ ripe Avocado
½ tsp. lime juice
1/8 diced tomato
6 crushed pistachios
Sea salt to taste
2 tsp. extra virgin oil

## Instructions

1. Toast the slice of keto bread.
2. Chop the avocado in half and sprinkle lime juice over it.
3. Place half of the avocado on top of the toast and smash it into the toast.
4. Sprinkle the crushed pistachios, diced tomatoes, and sea salt over the avocado and drizzle extra virgin oil over it.

5. Enjoy the healthy meal either with a knife.

***The amazing blend of avocados and pistachios not only offers an absolute delight but also adds an extra-healthy parameter to this lunch recipe. So, this keto toast makes a perfect lunch this season.***

## Lunch Recipe 2

## KETO EGGPLANT BURGER

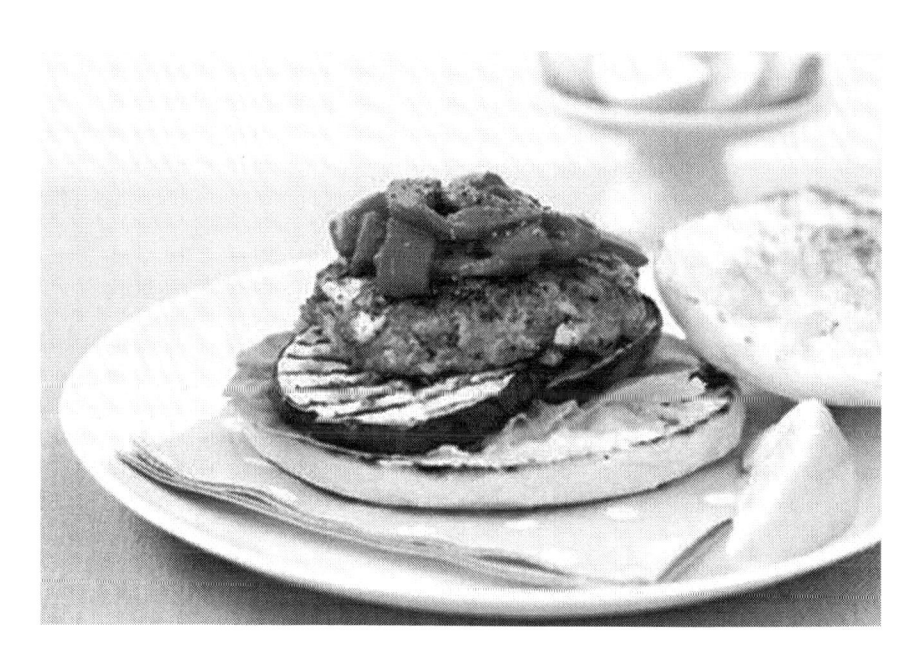

Nutritional value 376 cal
Protein 5 g
Fat 38 g
Carbohydrates 11 g

*A delicious lunch that is sure to become a prominent meal in your everyday life, this 'Keto Eggplant burger' features the freshness of eggplants with the delicious dipping sauce.*

Serves: 1
Preparation time: 10 minutes
Cooking time: 5 minutes

## Ingredients

### *For the eggplant burgers:*

½ lb. ground pork
2 small eggplants
2 small green onions, diced
1 tbsp. minced ginger
2 tbsp. gluten-free coconut aminos or tamari sauce
1 tsp. salt
Dash of pepper

### *For the dipping sauce:*

4 garlic cloves, minced
4 tbsp. gluten-free coconut aminos or tamari sauce
1 tsp. sesame oil
½ tsp. vinegar

## INSTRUCTIONS

1. Cut the two eggplants into thick slices of 1-inch each. Then, deliberately make small cuts through them to produce "burger buns" which are still hinged together.
2. Add the green onions, ground pork, tamari sauce, ginger, salt, and pepper in a large bowl and mix them together. Next, stuff this meat mixture into the "buns."
3. Allow them to steam for at least 20 minutes.

4. In order to make the dipping sauce, add the dipping sauce ingredients in a bowl and mix them together in a small bowl.
5. Enjoy the eggplant burgers with the dipping sauce.

***This keto eggplant burger recipe simply turns eggplant into a marvelous treat. It ensures you a full and satisfied meal, no matter what. Enjoy!***

## Lunch Recipe 3

## LOADED CAULIFLOWER BAKE

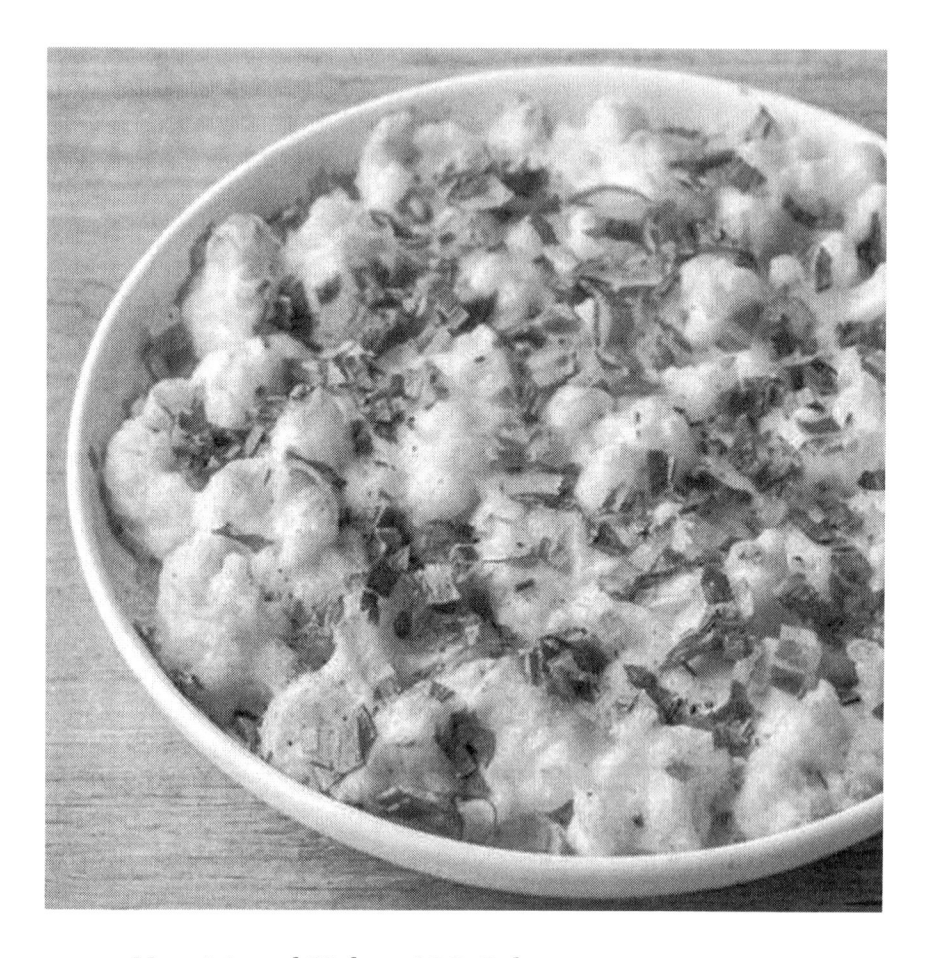

Nutritional Value 498 Cal
Protein 13.9 G
Fat 45 G
Carbohydrates 5.8 G

***No matter if you serve this easy and elegant cauliflower bakes with a bed of greens or with the***

*crumbled slices of bacon, it will quickly become your favorite recipe for lunch.*

Serves: 4
Preparation time: 5 minutes
Cooking time: 20 minutes

## Ingredients

1 large cauliflower head, cut into florets
1 cup heavy cream
2 tbsp. butter
2 oz. cream cheese
1 ¼ cup cheddar cheese, shredded and separated
Pinch salt and pepper to taste
6 cooked and crumbled slices of bacon
¼ cup green onions, chopped

## Instructions

1. Preheat the oven to 350 degrees.
2. Blanch cauliflower florets for 2-3 minutes in a large pot of boiling water. Remove cauliflower.
3. In a medium pot, add butter, cream cheese, heavy cream, 1 cup of cheddar cheese (shredded), and salt. Melt them together and combine well.
4. In a baking dish, add cheese sauce, cauliflower florets, 1 tbsp. crumbled bacon, and 1 tbsp. green onions. Stir them together.

5. Top with remaining crumbled bacon, shredded cheddar cheese, and green onions.
6. Bake in the oven until cheese turns golden and bubbly whereas cauliflower gets soft, for nearly 20 minutes.
7. Serve immediately and enjoy!

***This cauliflower recipe makes a perfect healthy lunch, as it requires handful of preparation and is ready to serve almost immediately. So get set for this dreamy lunch and enjoy!***

## Lunch Recipe 4

## LOW CARB KETO MEATLOAF

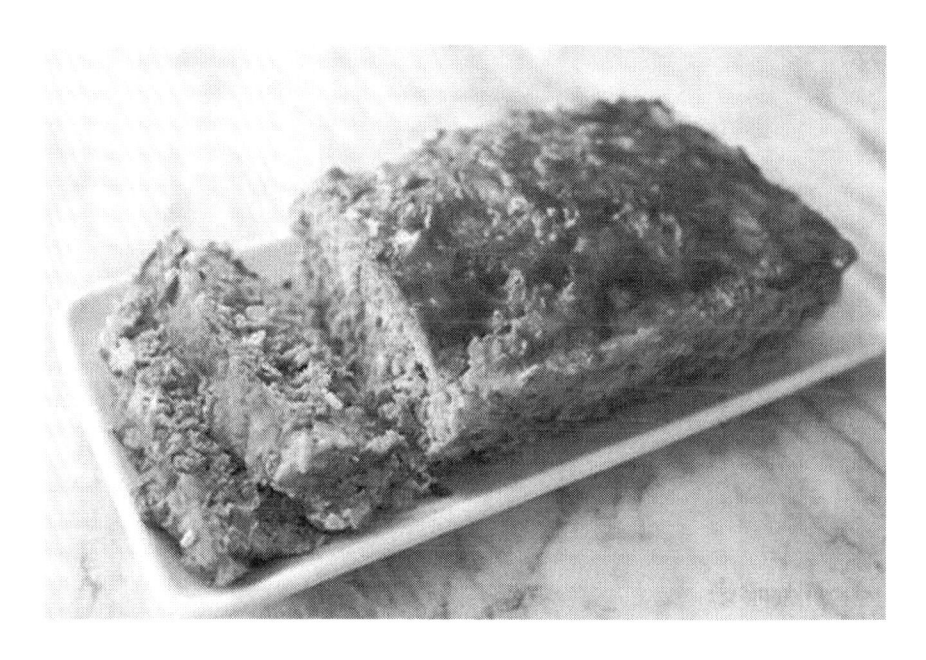

Nutritional value 344 cal
Protein 33 g
Fat 29 g
Carbohydrates 4 g

*If you are fond of the meatloaf, then this low carb keto meatloaf recipe is sure to cater to the same taste. All it takes is one pan to combine everything as instructed in the tutorial and you are ready with your healthy lunch within an hour.*

Serves: 6
Preparation time: 10 minutes
Cooking time: 50 minutes

## Ingredients

2 pounds ground beef (85% lean) (grass fed)
½ tbsp. salt
1 tsp. black pepper
¼ cup Nutritional Yeast
2 tbsp. avocado oil
2 large eggs
1 tbsp. lemon zest
¼ cup chopped fresh oregano
¼ cup chopped parsley
4 cloves garlic

## Instructions

1. Pre-heat oven to 400 F.
2. In a large bowl add ground beef, nutritional yeast, salt and black pepper and mix well.
3. In a blender add the eggs, herbs, garlic and oil. Blend until the lemon, herbs and garlic are minced whereas eggs are froth.
4. Add this egg blend to the beef mixture and combine well.
5. Next, add beef to an 8x4 loaf pan. Smooth it let it flatten out.
6. Bake in oven for an hour.
7. Remove from the oven and flop the loaf pan over the sink to do away with the fluid. Now, let it cool for 10 minutes before slicing into desired pieces.

8.     Garnish with fresh lemon and enjoy!

***This cauliflower recipe makes a perfect healthy lunch, as it requires handful of preparation and is ready to serve almost immediately. So get set for this dreamy lunch and enjoy!***

## Lunch Recipe 5

## CURRY CHICKEN LETTUCE WRAPS

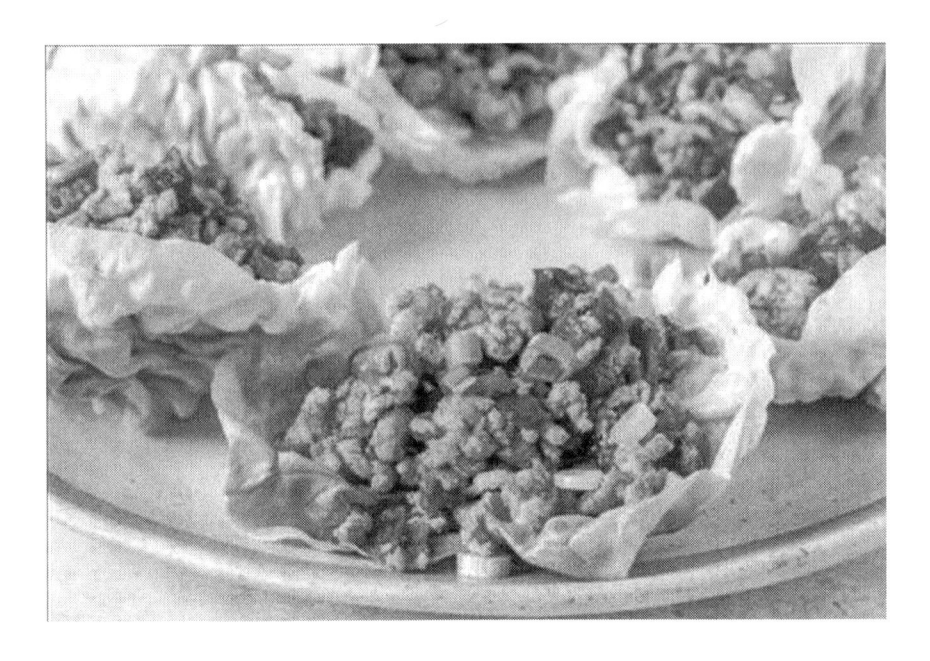

Nutritional value 554 cal
Protein 50 g
Fat 36 g
Carbohydrates 7 g

*Keto diets focus on grass-fed meats, and chicken is a great option for a low carb lunch. Give a tangy hint to your chicken, how about chicken wrapped in lettuce?*

Serves: 2
Preparation time: 5 minutes
Cooking time: 15 minutes

## Ingredients

1 lb. chicken thighs, boneless & skinless
¼ cup onion, minced
2 cloves of garlic, minced
2 tsp. Curry Powder
1 ½ tsp. salt
1 tsp. black pepper
3 tbsp. ghee
5-6 lettuce leaves
1 cup cauliflower rice
¼ cup sour cream, Lactose free or plain

## Instructions

1. Prepare your veggies and set them aside.
2. Chop your chicken thighs into 1-inch pieces each.
3. Next, bring a large skillet to boil. Add 2 tbsp. of ghee followed by the onion. Stir until browned.
4. Add the chicken, garlic and salt. Again, stir well.
5. Let the chicken be cooked until it turns brown in color, for about 8 minutes.
6. Now, stir in the last tablespoon of ghee, curry and the cauliflower rice. Sauté the mixture until well combined.
7. Lay out 5-6 lettuce leaves, and add curry chicken mixture into each one.
8. Serve the dish topped with a dollop of cream!

*This cuisine is a creamy yet tangy, you can serve this with zoodles as an optional method but it serves quite a meal itself.*

## Lunch Recipe 6

# LOW CARB HIGH FAT CHICKEN NUGGETS

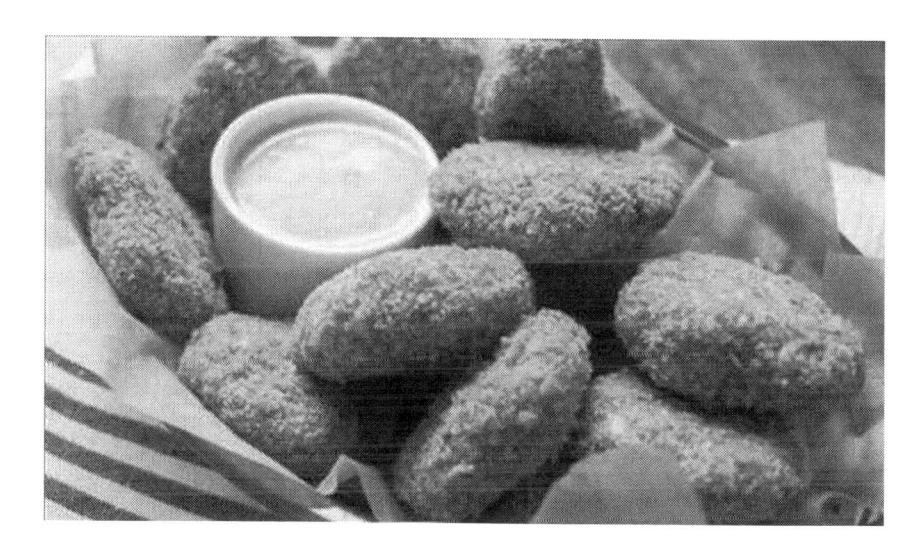

Nutritional value 443.2 cal
Protein 48 g
Fat 25 g
Carbohydrates 4 g

*Keto diets focus on grass-fed meats, and chicken is a great option for a low carb lunch. Give a tangy hint to your chicken, how about chicken nuggets?*

Serves: 2
Preparation time: 10 minutes
Cooking time: 15 minutes

## Ingredients

### First bowl

1 whisked egg
4 tbsp. oil of choice

### Second bowl

900 g chicken breast
100 g almond flour
½ tsp. salt
½ tsp. garlic powder
1 tsp. onion flakes

## Instructions

### First bowl

1. Using a fork, mix the oil and the eggs together.

### Second bowl

1. Mix the almond flour, garlic, salt and onion together.
2. Deliberately cut the chicken breasts into nuggets sized pieces. Dip each nugget in the first bowl and cover thoroughly with the coating.
3. Next, fry each chicken nugget in oil, until golden and cooked thoroughly on both the sides.
4. Enjoy with salsa, garlic mayo or sugar free tomato sauce.

*These chicken nuggets make a great lunch and sure to be your secret best friends. In fact the recipe has a great potential to make you fall in love with it. It is quite easy and convenient to prepare and doesn't require anything else to be a complete meal.*

## Lunch Recipe 8

### CHICKEN VEGETABLE SKILLET

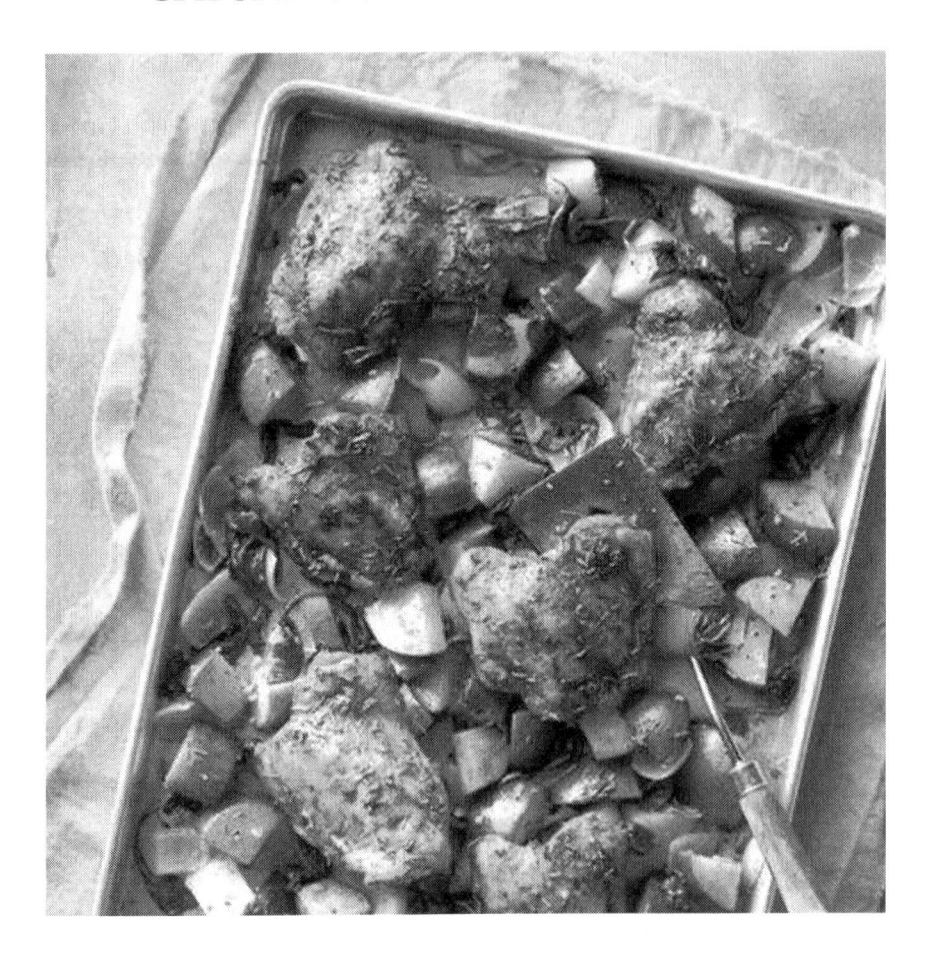

Serves: 2
Preparation time: 5 minutes
Cooking time: 20 minutes

***Keto diets focus on grass-fed meats, and chicken is a great option for a low carb lunch. Give a tangy***

*hint to your chicken, how about chicken veggie skillet?*

## Ingredients

2 tablespoons seasoned bread crumbs
1/2 pound boneless skinless chicken breast, cut into 1-inch strips
2 teaspoons canola oil, divided
1 small onion, chopped
1/2 cup sliced fresh carrot
1 small zucchini, sliced
1 small yellow summer squash, sliced
2 garlic cloves, minced
1/4 teaspoon pepper
1/8 teaspoon salt
2 tablespoons shredded cheese

## Instructions

1. First and foremost, keep the bread crumbs in a medium to large resalable plastic bag.
2. Gradually add on the chicken and shake thoroughly to help it coat on the bread crumbs.
3. Cook chicken in a large skillet coated with cooking spray, utilizing 1 teaspoon oil, over medium to high heat or until the juices are evidently running.
4. Remove the mixture and ensure it remains warm.

5. Sauté onion and carrot in the same skillet, using the remaining oil until it turns crispier and tenderer.
6. Introduce the zucchini, garlic squash, pepper and salt and bring them to boil for another 5 minutes or until vegetables are tender.
7. Take the chicken back to pan and sprinkle with cheese.

*This chicken skillet make a great lunch and sure to be your secret best friends. In fact the recipe has a great potential to make you fall in love with it. It is quite easy and convenient to prepare and doesn't require anything else to be a complete meal.*

## Lunch Recipe 8

## KETO HAM SPINACH MINI QUICHE

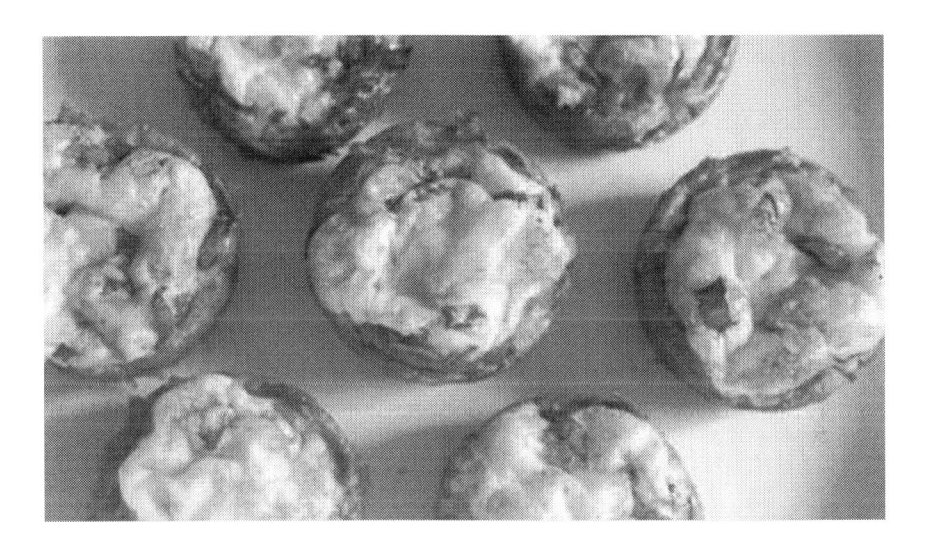

Nutritional value 443.2 cal
Protein 48 g
Fat 25 g
Carbohydrates 4 g

*This meal not only focuses on low carb diet, but is also the best way to have a delicious meal without compromising on your keto-diet routine. So, embrace yourself and start your afternoon with this keto ham spinach quiche.*

Serves: 2
Preparation time: 10 minutes
Cooking time: 15 minutes

## Ingredients

- 3 whisked eggs
- 4 diced slices of ham
- ¾ cup of chopped spinach
- ¼ cup chopped leek
- ¼ cup coconut milk
- ½ tsp. baking powder
- Pinch of salt and pepper to taste

## Instructions

1. Preheat oven to 350 F.
2. In a large mixing bowl, add whisked eggs, chopped spinach, diced ham, chopped leek, baking powder, coconut milk, salt and pepper and mix well.
3. Distribute the mixture evenly into 4 tart pans or small mini quiche.
4. Bake the mixture for 15 minutes in the oven.
5. Serve as a delicious lunch or a quick snack.

**This amazing ham mini quiche has earned itself the reputation of bringing huge smiles on faces, so no matter if you have to throw a house party to your loved ones or a little bash with your partner, this keto recipe will never disappoint you.**

# Lunch Recipe 9

## PEACH PAN FRIED SCALLOPS SALAD RECIPE

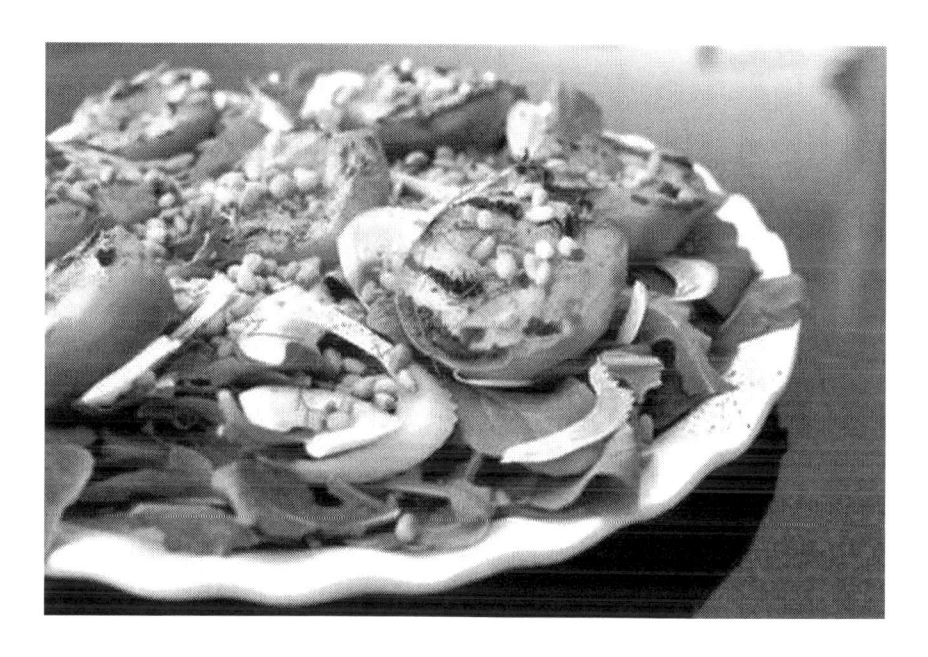

Nutritional value 130 cal
Protein 48 g
Fat 8 g
Carbohydrates 7 g

*What makes this marvellously elaborate recipe a pure treat is its ketogenic nature. Get ready with your frying pan, as this good afternoon recipe is not only* easy to prepare and amazing to eat, but also makes a perfect lunch idea if you were ever to throw a treat to a crowd!

Serves: 2
Preparation time: 5 minutes
Cooking time: 10 minutes

## Ingredients

12 small scallops (About 90 grams)
Coconut oil
5 oz. arugula leaves
½ sliced onion
1 sliced peach
1 tsp. oil
1 tsp. lemon juice

## Instructions

1. In a frying pan, add coconut oil.
2. Add scallops to the pan and fry for at least 5 minutes on both sides.
3. Toss the onion slices, arugula, peach slices, lemon juice and olive oil together.
4. Serve the scallops after placing them on tops of the salad.

***Quick and easy scallop salad recipe, it is low carb and is easy and quick meal to make. We recommend you to double the delight of the recipe by sharing it with your loved ones as a great lunch.***

## Lunch Recipe 10

### CHICKEN TERIYAKI

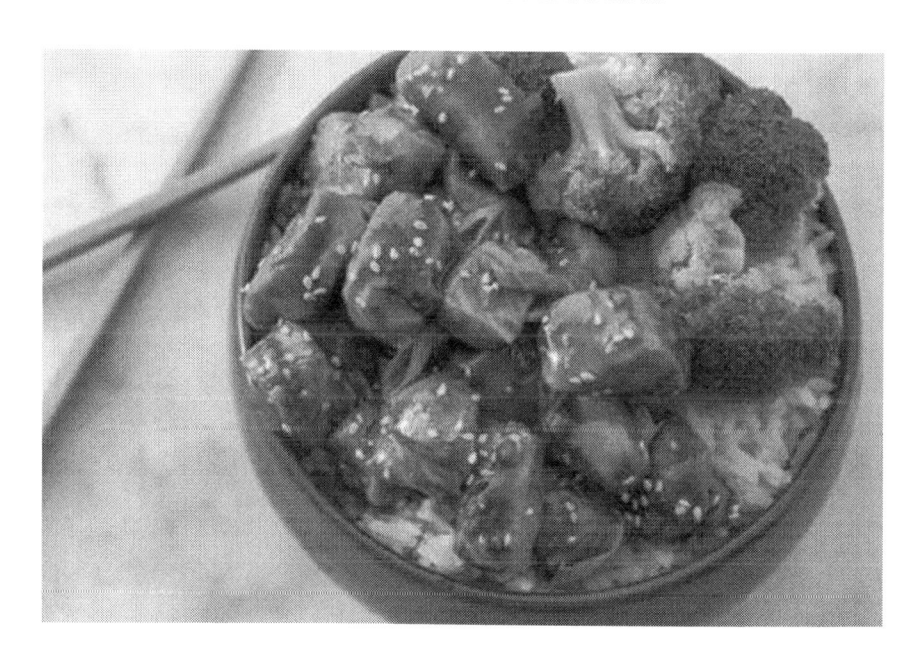

Nutritional value 342 cal
Protein 52 g
Fat 7 g
Carbohydrates 12 g

*The fusion of chicken and teriyaki sauce is not only taste-full, but also takes this recipe to the pinnacle of deliciousness. So, the Keto Chicken Teriyaki makes a perfectly healthy treat this fall.*

Serves: 2
Preparation time: 10 minutes
Cooking time: 20 minutes

## Ingredients

1 ½ lbs chicken thigh skin on-2 pieces
Salt to taste
½ tbsp ghee / oil to pan fry the chicken
Toasted white sesame seeds (optional)

### *Teriyaki Sauce*

2 ½ tbsp coconut aminos
1 tbsp ginger garlic paste
1 tbsp apple cider vinegar
¾ tbsp red boat fish sauce

## Instructions

1. Heat 1/2 tbsp ghee over medium/high heat. When hot, add chicken. Skin side down. Pan Fry about 10 minutes until the skin is crispy.
2. Flip and pan fry the other side until the chicken is completely cooked through.
3. Drain the extra oil and keep the chicken aside.
4. **Make the sauce:** In the same sauce pan, add all the ingredients of the teriyaki sauce mentioned above and heat the pan over medium heat.
5. When the sauce is thickened, add the chicken to it. Coat the saucer over the chicken well.
6. Add white sesame seeds and let the chicken absorb the sauce.

## For Garnish

1. Wait for 5 minutes before serving, when cooled down serve with rice.

*This makes a great recipe for the coming holidays! Get set to give it all to your friends and family at Christmas time. But remember: Do not allow the balls sit in the chocolate for long or they might just melt.*

## Lunch Recipe 11

# ASIAN CHICKEN AND CABBAGE SALAD

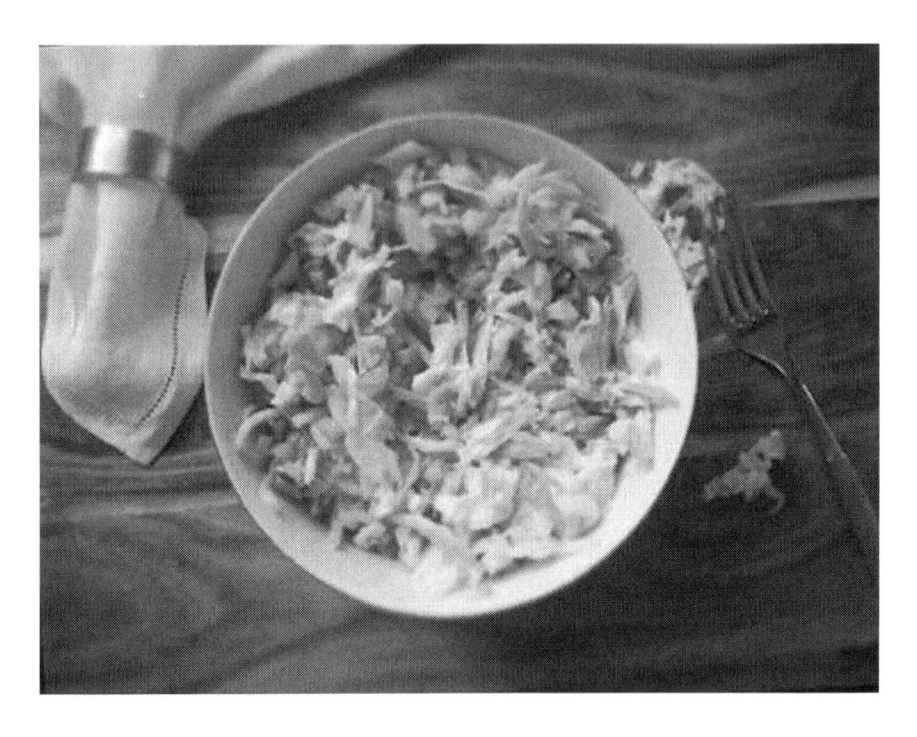

Nutritional value 227.2 cal
Protein 16.4 g
Fat 15.3 g
Carbohydrates 5.9 g

*For those days when you really want to cook their heart out and go for a heavier option than just lighter salads for lunch, go for this creamy chicken recipe!*

Serves: 2
Total time 30 minutes

## Ingredients

½ head green cabbage, shredded
1 boneless, skinless chicken breasts
½ tsp olive oil
¼ cup of avocado oil
½ large shallot
3 cloves garlic, chopped
½ tbsp lime juice
½ tbsp fish sauce
½ tsp salt, more to taste
¼ tsp white pepper
½ tsp coconut palm sugar
½ tsp apple cider vinegar
2 carrots
1 spicy red chile pepper, seeds removed and thinly sliced
1/2 small handful cilantro leaves, coarsely chopped
1/2 small handful mint leaves, coarsely chopped

## Instructions

1. Take a large ball and place the shredded cabbage inside it.
2. This bowl needs to be filled with cold water.
3. Add little bit of salt to it and stir to combine. Set aside to soak for 20 minutes.
4. While the cabbage is soaking in the water, grill the chicken. Carefully rub the chicken breast all

over using olive oil. Dress with a bit of salt and pepper according to taste.
5. Add the chicken on the hot grill and let it cook for about 6 minutes, flipping every couple of minutes.
6. Get ready with a bowl of ice water and shift the cooked chicken to equip it for the ice water bath. Set it aside to be cooled for at least 5 minutes.
7. While the chicken is again busy soaking, you can heat the avocado oil in a pan over high heat. Now, bring the shallots and boil until they turn translucent, for at least 2 minutes. Add the garlic.
8. Stir-fry the recipe until it attains a golden color, while stirring regularly to evade scorching, for nearly 3 more minutes.
9. Add the oil into a medium sized bowl via a strainer, while catching the shallots and garlic to drain; save the oil and allow it to cool for 5 minutes.
10. When the oil gets enough cool, mix it together with the lime juice, salt, fish sauce, white pepper, apple cider vinegar, coconut palm sugar to make the dressing.
11. Shred the chicken together with the grain, by making use of the forks, and setting them aside.

12. Remove the cabbage and let it dry with paper towels.
13. In a large bowl, mix the chicken, cabbage, carrots, cilantro, Chile pepper, mint, and the salad dressing.
14. Toss the ingredients to combine. Add salt according to taste, then serve topped with the fried shallots and garlic.

**This is a smart salad which pleases most of the people following KETO diets. A little tricky to conduct the procedure but a tasty dish awaits behind all that hard work.**

# Lunch Recipe 12

## CHICKEN TACO SALAD

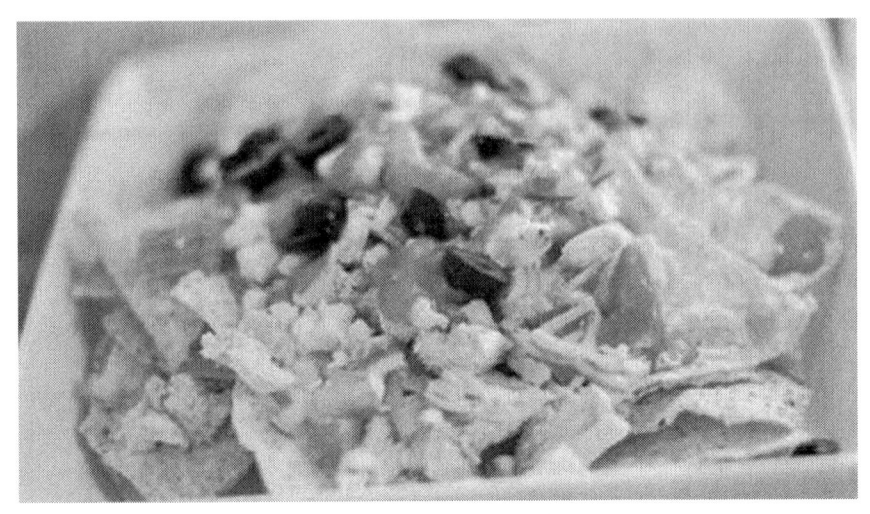

Image source: The pioneer Woman

Nutritional value 270 cal
Protein 20 g
Fat 18 g
Carbohydrates 14 g

*This lunch recipe couldn't have met a simpler and more convenient fate. Made from the wholesome and delicious ingredients, this KETO chicken taco salad is best eaten fresh, so get set for this health-studded paradise.*

## Ingredients

2 boneless and skinless chicken breasts
2 cups of romaine lettuce

1 diced tomato
½ diced avocado
½ diced bell pepper
¼ cup of mayonnaise, homemade
2 tbsp of olive oil;
2 tbsp of lime juice;
¼ cup finely chopped cilantro

***For taco seasoning***

1 tbsp. of chili powder
¼ tsp. of garlic powder;
1 tsp. of ground cumin;
¼ tsp. of onion powder;
¼ tsp. of red pepper flakes;
¼ tsp. of oregano;
¼ tsp. of paprika;
Sea salt to taste
Freshly ground black pepper to taste

## Instructions

1. Get the grill ready by pre-heating at medium-high.
2. Combine the ingredients for the taco seasoning.
3. Stroke the chicken using half of the taco seasoning.
4. Add the chicken to the preheated grill.
5. Cook the chicken for 10 to 12 minutes, turning if needed.
6. Let the chicken cool down and then cut it into cubes.

7. Add the mayo, olive oil, lime juice, and the other half of the taco seasoning in a small bowl.
8. Toss the lettuce, tomatoes, avocado and bell pepper in a large sized bowl.
9. Dress the salad using the chicken and sprinkle dressing on top.
10. Serve with cilantro topped.

**The lettuce, tomatoes, avocado and bell pepper add vibrancy and show off the nutrients within this colorful salad. For picky eaters you can add the contents into separate bowl.**

## Lunch Recipe 13

## SMOKED SALMON KETO WRAP

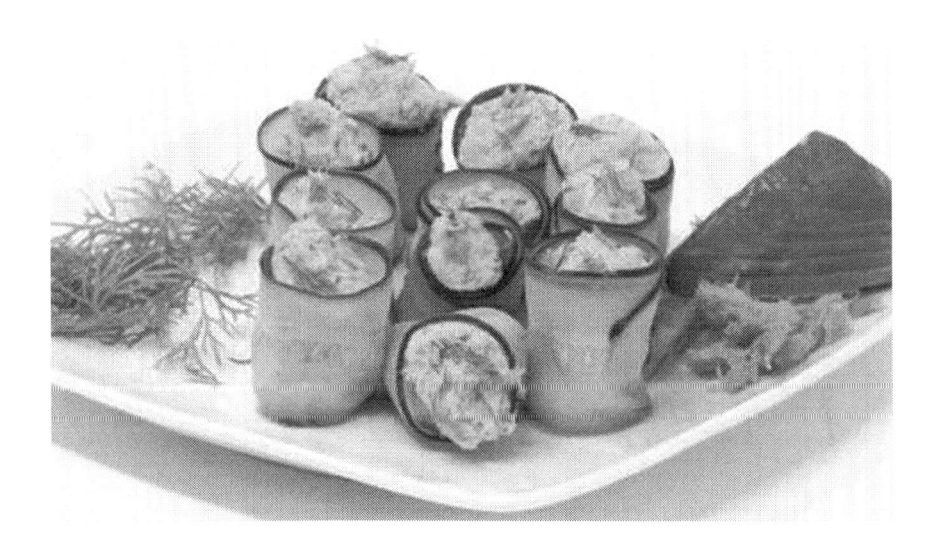

Nutritional value 210 cal
Protein 29 g
Fat 10 g
Carbohydrates 0 g

*This good noon smoked salmon wraps not only focus on low carb diet, but also serve the pinnacle of delight to your taste buds. So, sit back and relax, your afternoon is all set to be enlightened by this keto wrap.*

Serves: 2
Preparation time: 5 minutes
Cooking time: 0 minutes

## Ingredients

4 Ham Slices
½ cucumber, cut into thin slices
3.5 oz. smoked salmon
1 tbsp. coconut cream
Green salad for serving

## Instructions

1. Evenly distribute coconut cream on each of the four hams.
2. On the top of each ham slice, place a slice of smoked salmon.
3. Next, place thin slices of cucumber on the top of each salmon topped ham.
4. Now, roll the wrap up. Place the wrap on top of the green salad before serving.

*A quick and easy recipe, it is low carb and is easy and quick meal to make. We recommend you to double the delight of the recipe by sharing it with your loved ones as a great lunch.*

## Lunch Recipe 14

### GARLICKY KETO GREENS

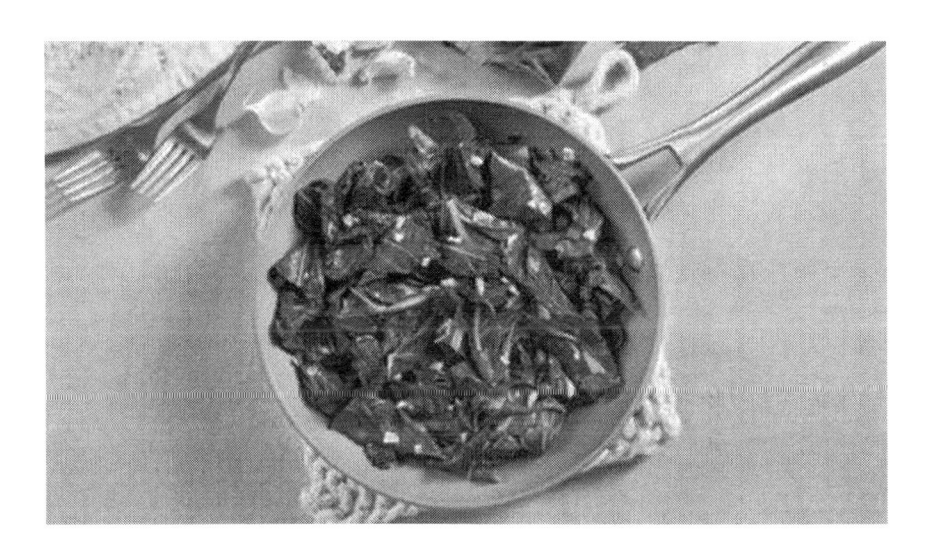

Nutritional value 190 cal
Protein 3 g
Fat 16 g
Carbohydrates 10 g

*These taste-studded Garlicky greens rock the demands in the restaurants, thanks to their healthy yet delicious nature. It's not only keto, but also assures you of its healthy features by simply being Whole 30 and lower carb.*

Serves: 2
Preparation time: 5 minutes
Cooking time: 10 minutes

## Ingredients

Collard greens, 1 bunch
4-6 garlic cloves
1/3 tsp. of sea salt, for taste
2 tbsp. coconut oil or extra virgin olive oil

## Instructions

1. Clean and rinse the collard leaves and let them dry.
2. Use a knife to cut them in a V shape through center of the stem. Then proceed to cut leaf in half.
3. Hold together 6 leaf halves and tightly roll them up.
4. Cut the strips crosswise in a way that they are quarter inch wide.
5. Next, try to cut the slimmer strips in half making sure that one remains long lengthwise.
6. Continue the above steps until all leaves are cut into strips.
7. Next, heat the oil in a medium size pan and heat for at least 1 minute.
8. Now, bring in garlic and salt together and keep boiling till garlic turns fragrant, for nearly 2 minutes.
9. Bring in collard strips and sauté them while stirring frequently, until they turn bright in color and soften up. Watch them carefully to

avoid overcooking. It should ideally take around 6-8 minutes.
10. Serve immediately and enjoy!

***This meal serves multiple purposes by focusing on low carb and gluten free diet. So, embrace yourself and gift yourself this dreamy lunch.***

# Lunch Recipe 15

## KETO FISH STICKS

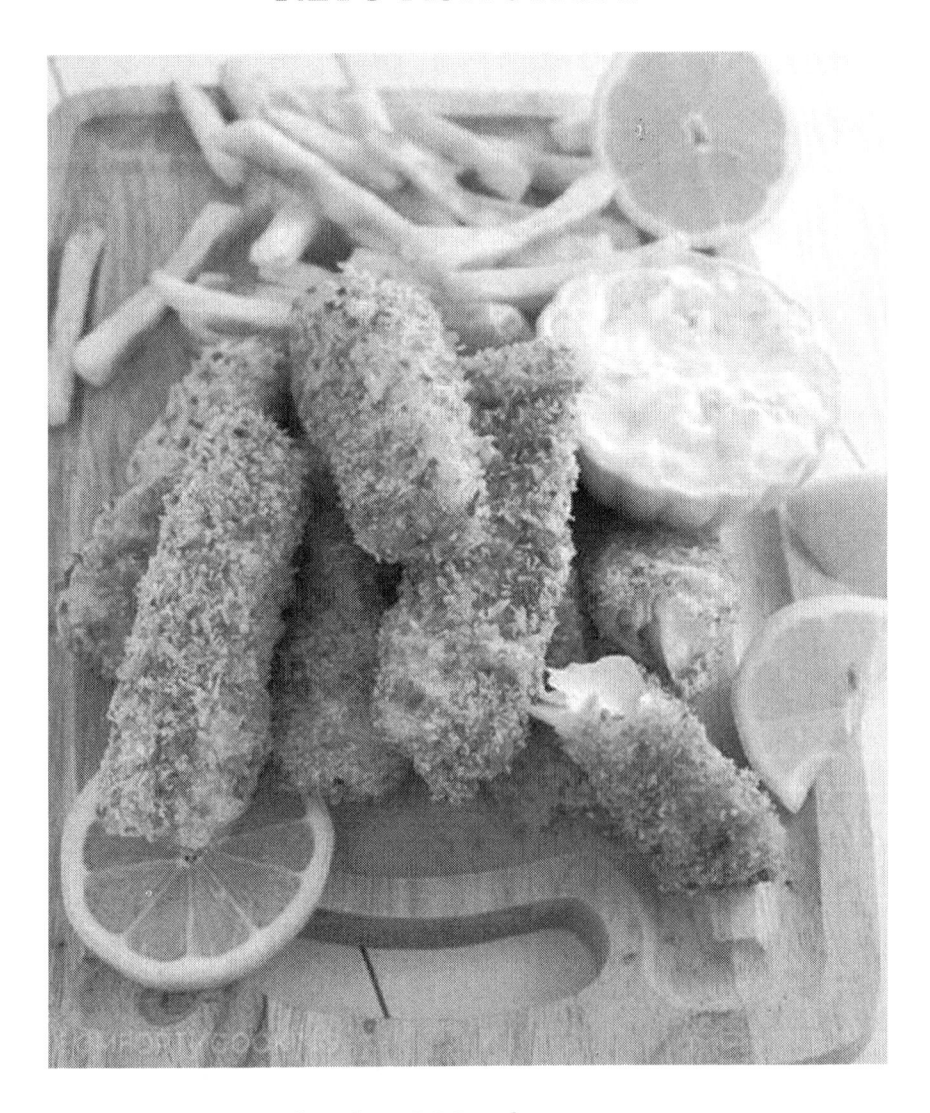

Nutritional value 289 cal
Protein 39 g
Fat 12 g
Carbohydrates 1 g

*If you think fish sticks cannot be healthy then you are yet to come across this magician dish. Served as a typical keto lunch, it will soon take over the place of your favourite recipe.*

Serves: 3
Preparation time: 10 minutes
Cooking time: 15 minutes

## Ingredients

3.5 oz. Pork Rinds, crush in food processor
10 oz. Fresh Cod fillet, cut into strips
1 tbsp. coconut flour
½ tsp. black pepper
¼ tsp. sea salt
1 large egg
1 tsp. of water

## Instructions

1. Preheat your oven to 400 degrees F.
2. In a medium bowl, add coconut flour, fish strips, and spices. Mix with your hands until well coated. Set aside.
3. Place the crushed pork rinds in a paper bag and set aside.
4. Whisk the eggs one by one in a large bowl full of water. Now, dip the fish strips one after the other in this egg mixture and places them in the paper bag with the pork rinds. Shake well to coat.

5. Next, place the fish strips on a lightly greased baking sheet and bake in the preheated oven for 15 minutes.
6. Remove from oven and serve.

***Just when you were bored of the typical lunch recipes, these keto fish sticks paved their way to our recipe book and came to your health and taste bud's rescue. Enjoy a rich blend of taste and health with this amazing recipe and thank us later.***

# Lunch Recipe 16

## SMOKY TUNA PICKLE BOATS

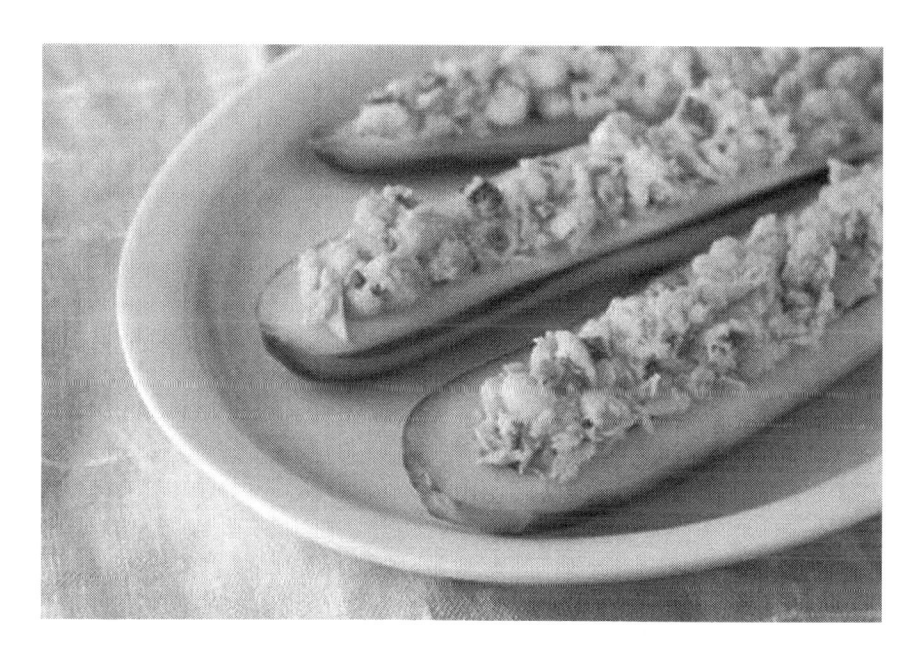

Nutritional value 118 cal
Protein 11 g
Fat 7 g
Carbohydrates 1.5 g

***This is a Quick and Easy to prepare keto lunch that is enriched with the goodness of tuna. Jam packed with the deliciousness, these tuna boats are relatively quick to be served as a lunch.***

Serves: 3
Preparation time: 10 minutes
Cooking time: 0 minutes

## Ingredients

Two 6 oz. cans albacore tuna
One 6 oz. can smoked tuna
1/3 cup mayo (sugar-free)
½ tsp. onion powder or 1 tbsp. dehydrated onion flakes
6 medium whole dill pickles
¼ tsp. garlic powder
¼ tsp. ground black pepper

## Instructions

1. In a medium sized bowl, add all the ingredients except for pickle and mix well.
2. Deliberately cut the pickles into half and scoop out the seeds from the middle.
3. Spoon nearly 3 tbsp. tuna salad into each pickle half.
4. Refrigerate overnight and serve.

*This delicious tuna boat recipe is loaded with the goodness of a rich color, incorporated with healthy ingredient, thus making it a high protein and low carb meal.*

## Lunch Recipe 17

## KETO CORN DOG MUFFINS

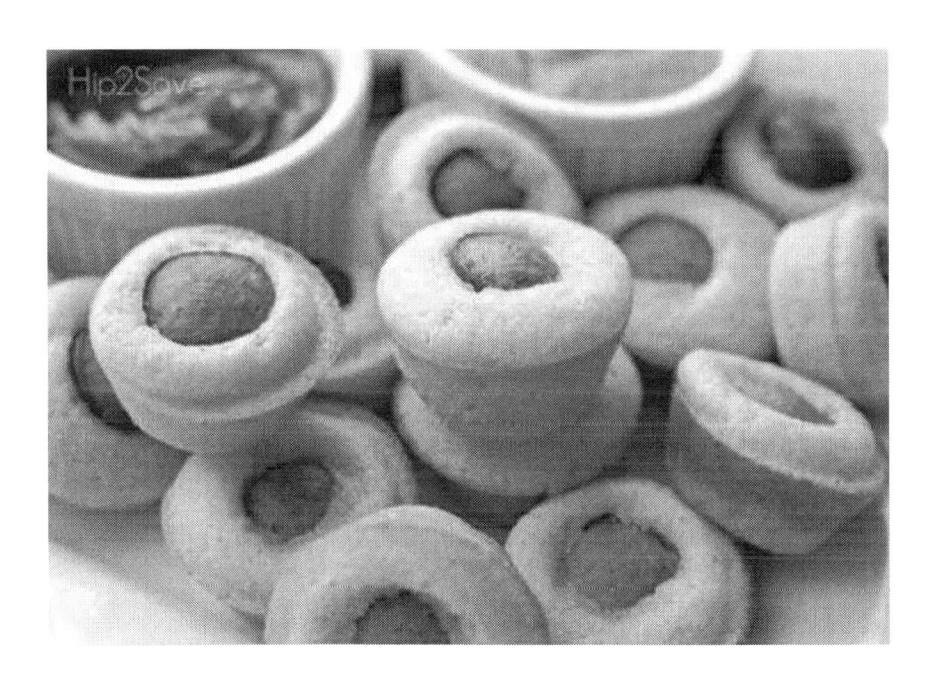

Nutritional value 159 cal
Protein 6 g
Fat 13 g
Carbohydrates 4 g

*An easy to prepare, healthy to eat, and amazingly addicting Keto dog muffin recipe, it is a simply perfect lunch idea if you were ever to throw a treat to a crowd! This recipe is perfectly Soy-free, Mayo-free, Whole 30 friendly and perfectly paleo.*

Serves: 1
Preparation time: 10 minutes
Cooking time: 25 minutes

## Ingredients

- 6 Eggs
- 10 organic hot dogs
- 1 cup Coconut Milk
- 4 tbsp. melted butter
- 4 tbsp. melted coconut oil
- 1 cup coconut flour
- 1 cup almond flour
- ½ tsp. salt for taste
- 1 tsp. Baking Soda

## Instructions

1. Preheat oven to 350 degree F.
2. Slice the hotdogs and set them aside.
3. Melt coconut oil and butter.
4. In a large mixing bowl, add almond flour, coconut flour, baking soda, eggs, oil, and butter. Combine all these ingredients and mix well.
5. Next, add hot dogs and coconut milk to the batter and mix together until the batter is light and fluffy.
6. Place baking cups in a muffin pan and equally fill with batter.
7. Bake in the preheated oven for 20-25 minutes.
8. Serve with mustard, mayo and sugar-free ketchup.

## Lunch Recipe 18

# SLOW COOKER GARLIC CHIPOTLE LIME CHICKEN

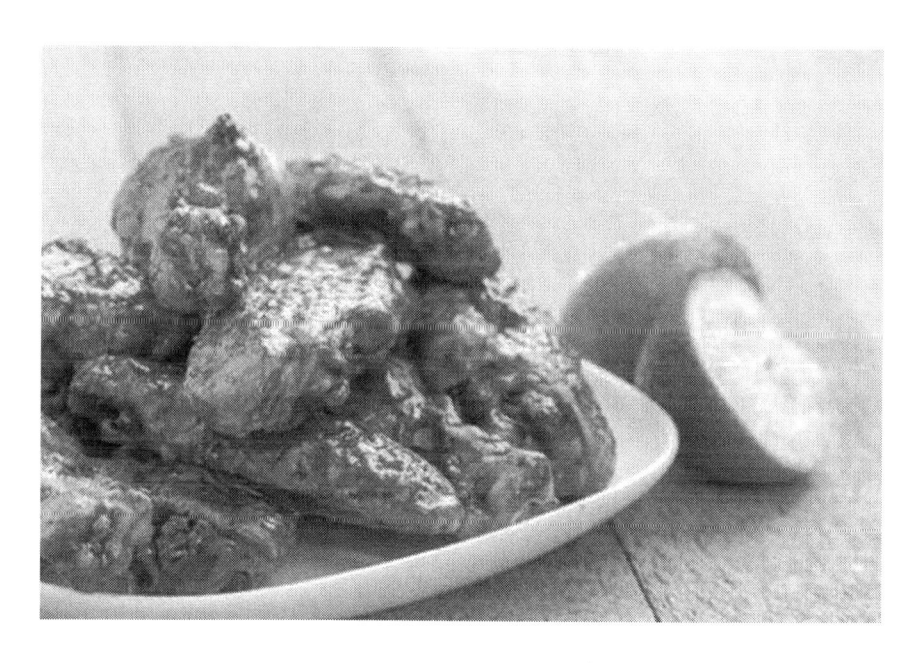

Nutritional value 183 cal
Protein 22 g
Fat 9 g
Carbohydrates 2 g

*As keto-diets focus on grass-fed meats a lot, chicken is a great option for lunch. Give a tangy hint to your chicken, how about chicken tossed in lemon!*

Serves: 6
Preparation time: 6 minutes
Cooking time: 5 hours

## Ingredients

1 ½ lb. chicken thighs or breasts, boneless and skinless

***Sauce Ingredients:***

⅓ Cup tomato sauce
2 tbsp. avocado oil or olive oil
2-3 cloves of garlic
2 tbsp. canned green chilies
1 tbsp. apple cider vinegar
3 tbsp. lime juice
⅓ cups flat leaf Italian parsley or fresh cilantro
1 ½ tsp. sweetener of choice
1 tsp. ground chipotle powder
1 tsp. sea salt for taste
¼ tsp. black pepper for taste

## Instructions

1. Add all the sauce ingredients in a food processor and pulse until a smooth batter forms.
2. Add chicken thighs or breasts in a slow cooker and cook on low or high heat.
3. Pour over the sauce at the top of chicken, close the lid of the slow cooker and cook for at least 5 hours on high. Serve & enjoy.

*The combination of chicken wingers and the exotic sauce makes a great lunch and sure to be your secret best friends. In fact the combination has a great potential to make you fall in love with it. The recipe is quite easy and convenient to prepare and doesn't require anything else to be a complete meal.*

## Lunch Recipe 19

# FRESH SRIRACHA BROCCOLI SALAD

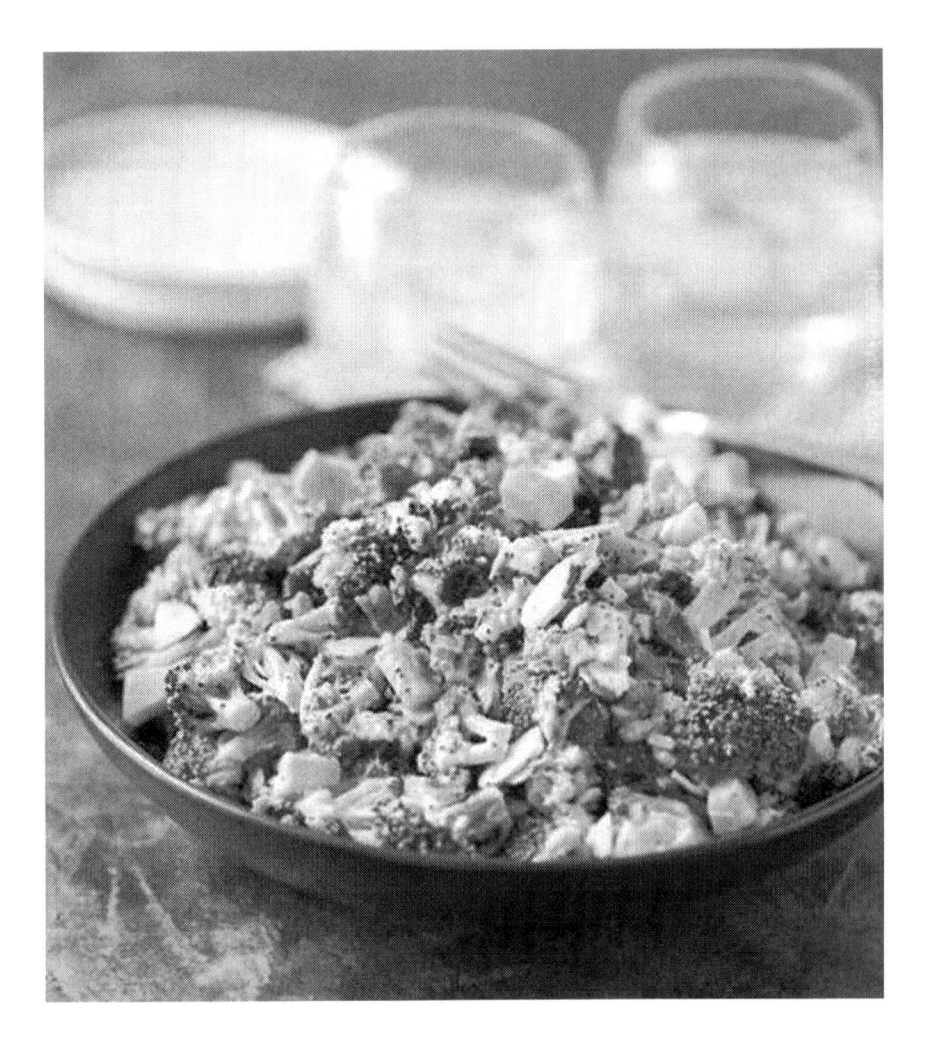

Nutritional value 212 cal
Protein 10 g
Fat 16 g
Carbohydrates 9 g

*An easy to prepare, healthy to eat, and amazingly addicting sriracha broccoli salad is simply a perfect lunch idea if you were ever to throw a treat to a crowd! This recipe is perfectly Soy-free, Mayo-free, Whole 30 friendly and perfectly Keto.*

Serves: 4
Preparation Time: 5 minutes
Cooking Time: 0 hours

## Ingredients

1 large head of broccoli, chopped
½ red bell pepper, sliced into 1/4" bites
1 cup mayonnaise
½ cup cheddar cheese, shredded
¼ cup salted sunflower seeds (dry, roasted)
6 slices of baked and crumbled bacon
½ tbsp. apple cider vinegar
1/3 tbsp. sriracha sauce
Pinch Salt and freshly grounded black pepper

## Instructions

1. In a large bowl, add all the ingredients and mix well.
2. Store the mixture in a sealed container for at least an hour and then enjoy!

*The amazing blend of sriracha, broccoli and other veggies in a salad not only offers an absolute delight but also adds an extra-healthy parameter to this salad.*

## Lunch Recipe 20

## KETO CHICKEN ENCHILADA BOW

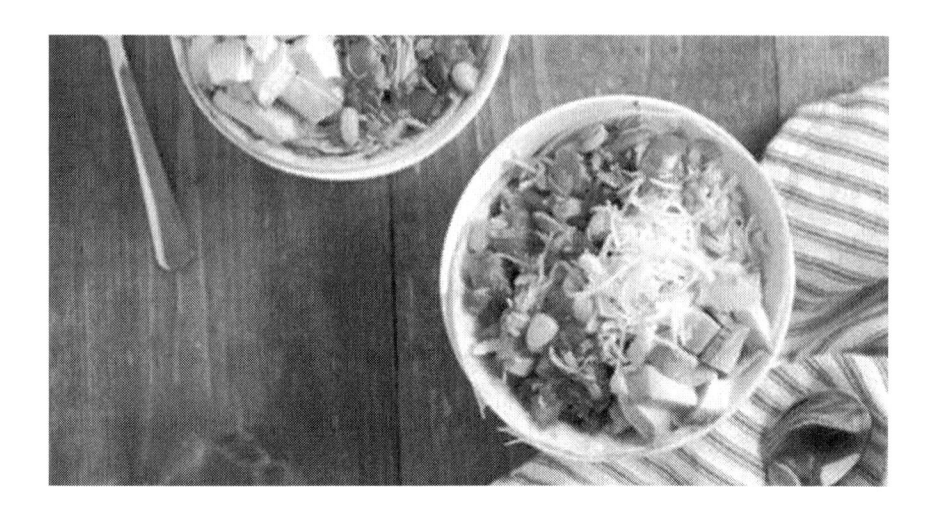

Nutritional value 120 cal
Protein 1 g
Fat 6 g
Carbohydrates 2 g

*This good noon chicken enchilada bowls not only focuses on low carb diet, but also Serves: the pinnacle of delight to your taste buds. So, sit back and relax, your afternoon is all set to be enlightened by this enchilada bowl.*

Serves: 6
Preparation time: 5 minutes
Cooking time: 20 minutes

## Ingredients

- 2-3 chicken breasts or 1 pound chicken
- ¾ cups red enchilada sauce
- ¼ cup onion
- ¼ cup water
- One 4 oz. can of green chills
- One 12 oz. steam bag full of cauliflower rice
- Preferred toppings- Avocado, cheese, avocado, jalapeno, and tomatoes
- Seasoning of choice for taste

## Instructions

1. Cook chicken breasts in a skillet over low-medium heat until lightly brown.
2. Add chilies, enchilada sauce, onions and water, and reduce heat to simmer. Cover the skillet.
3. Cook until chicken is completely cooked and then shred it.
4. Add the chicken back into the sauce and simmer for another 10 minutes uncovered or till the liquid had dried out.
5. Get the cauliflower rice prepared as per the instructions on the packaging and dice with preferred toppings
6. Top rice with chicken, avocado, cheese or preferred toppings

***This amazing enchilada bowl has long known for pleasing the crowd, so no matter if you have to***

*throw a house party to your loved ones or a little bash with your partner, this Keto recipe will never disappoint you.*

## Lunch Recipe 21

## KETO BROCCOLI BEEF RECIPE

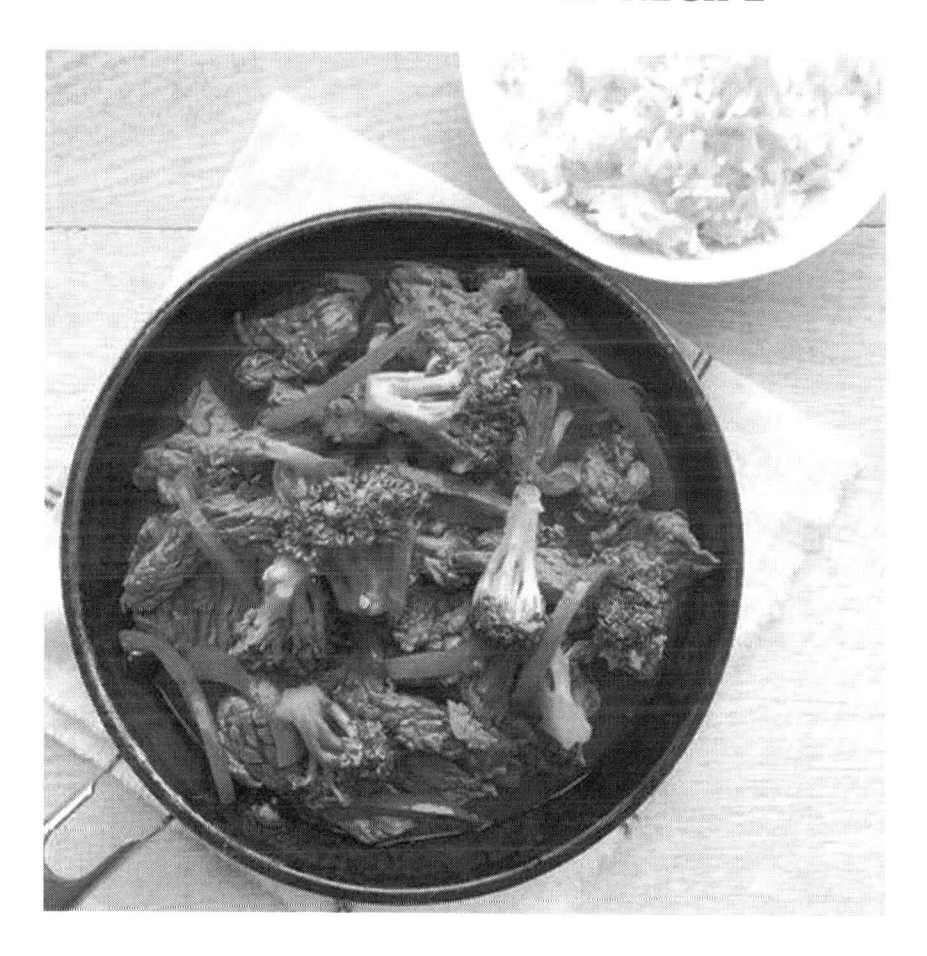

Nutritional value 152 cal
Protein 11 g
Fat 8 g
Carbohydrates 5 g

*What makes this marvellously elaborate recipe a pure treat is its gluten-free nature. Get ready with your skillets, as this good afternoon recipe is not only easy to prepare and amazing to eat, but also makes a perfect lunch idea if you were ever to throw a treat to a crowd!*

Serves: 2
Preparation time: 5 minutes
Cooking time: 15 minutes

## Ingredients

8 oz. broccoli florets
½ lb. beef, thinly sliced and precooked
3 garlic cloves, crushed
1 tsp. ginger, freshly grated
2 tbsp. coconut aminos
Coconut oil to cook in

## Instructions

1. In a skillet, add 2 tbsp. coconut oil and bring it to a boil. Next, add the broccoli florets.
2. When the broccoli gets tender, stir in the beef.
3. Saute' for a couple of minutes and then add in the ginger, garlic, and coconut aminos.
4. Serve immediately.

*This quick and easy lunch recipe is keto in nature and is easy and quick meal to make. We recommend you to double the delight of the recipe by sharing it with your loved ones as a great lunch.*

## Lunch Recipe 22

# GARLIC ROASTED SHRIMP WITH ZUCCHINI PASTA

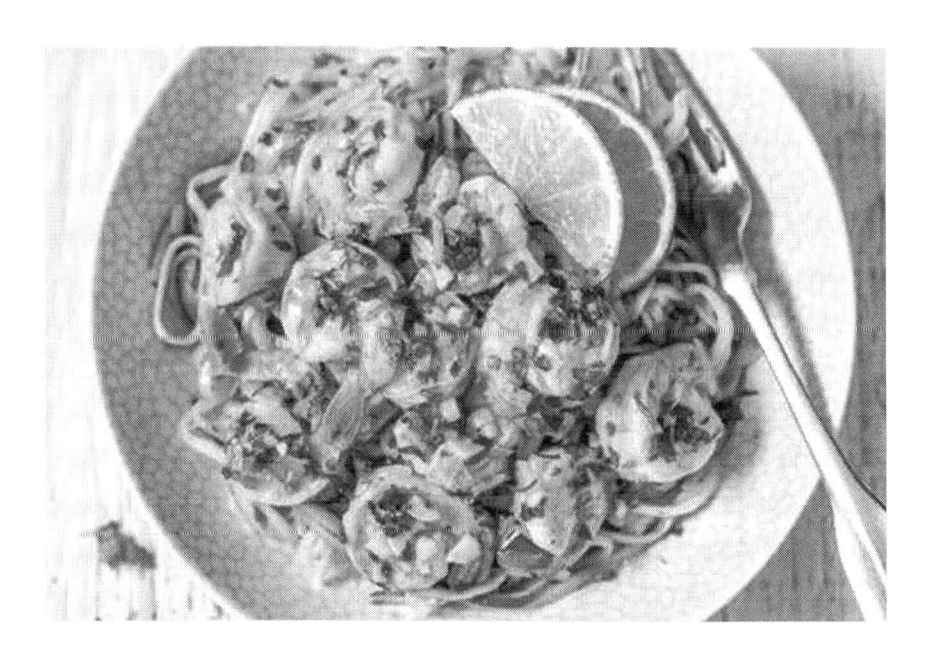

Nutritional value 409 cal
Protein 25 g
Fat 31 g
Carbohydrates 8 g

*Just when you were bored of the typical lunch recipes, this zucchini pasta paved its way to our recipe book and came to your health and taste bud's rescue. Enjoy a rich blend of taste and health with this amazing recipe and thank us later.*

Serves: 2
Preparation time: 10 minutes
Cooking time: 10 minutes

## Ingredients

8 ounces shrimp, peeled and deveined
2 tbsp. olive oil
2 tbsp. melted ghee or olive oil
2 minced garlic cloves
1 lemon, zested and juiced
¼ tsp. salt for taste
Freshly ground pepper to taste
2 medium zucchini sliced into thin strips for pasta

## Instructions

1. Preheat oven to 400 degrees.
2. Add all the ingredients in a baking dish and combine them well.
3. Bake in the preheated oven for 5-10 minutes or until shrimp turns pink in color.
4. Add the zucchini pasta, toss and serve.

# Lunch Recipe 23 (Dessert)

## CHOCOLATE ALMOND KETO FAT BOMB

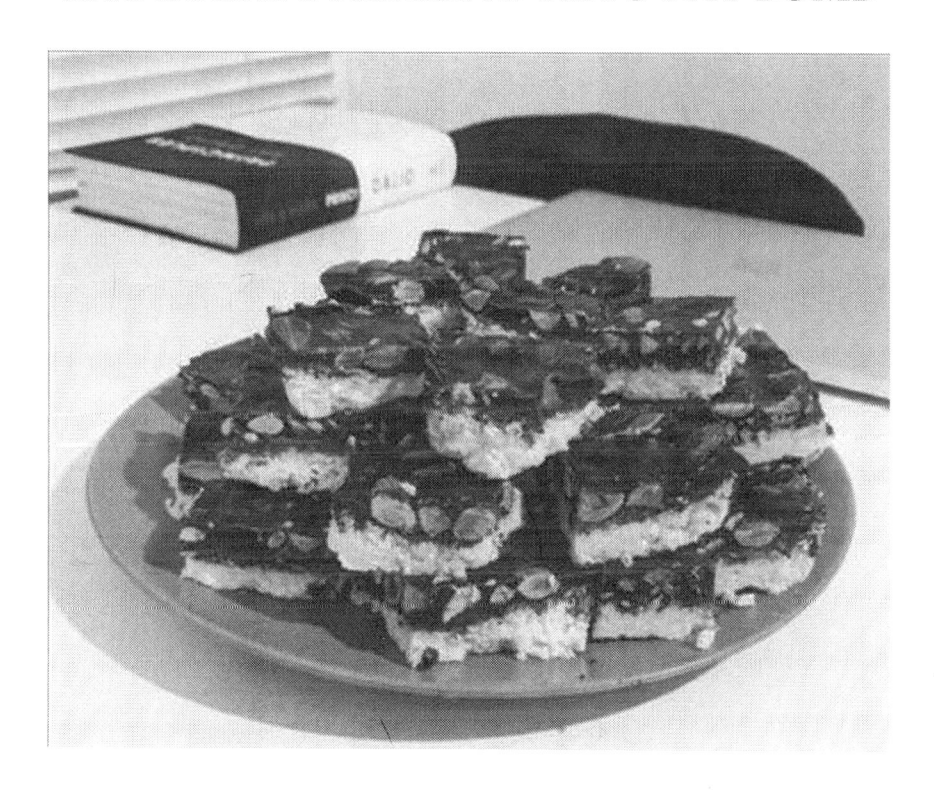

Nutritional value 131 cal
Protein 3 g
Fat 12 g
Carbohydrates 5 g

***What makes this marvellously elaborate dessert recipe a pure treat is its ketogenic nature. Get ready with your saucepans, as this good afternoon recipe is not only easy to prepare and amazing to eat, but also makes a perfect after-lunch dessert if you were ever to throw a treat to a crowd!***

Serves: 15
Preparation time: 5 minutes
Cooking time: 0 minutes

## Ingredients

1 cup Almond butter
1 cup Coconut Oil
½ cup Cacao Powder
¼ cup Coconut Flour
Stevia to taste
10-15 whole Almonds

## Instructions

1. In a small saucepan, melt coconut oil and almond butter. Add in the coconut flour, cacao powder, and stevia, and mix well.
2. Allow the mixture to become cool and then use your hands to shape 10-15 ping-pong sized balls from the mixture.
3. Deliberately stick an almond at the middle of each ball.
4. Let them refrigerate until you're ready to eat them.

*Quick and easy after-lunch dessert, these fat bombs are keto in nature and are easy and quick meal to make. We recommend you to double the delight of the recipe by sharing it with your loved ones as a great lunch.*

# Lunch Recipe 24 (Dessert)

## KETO MACAROON FAT BOMBS

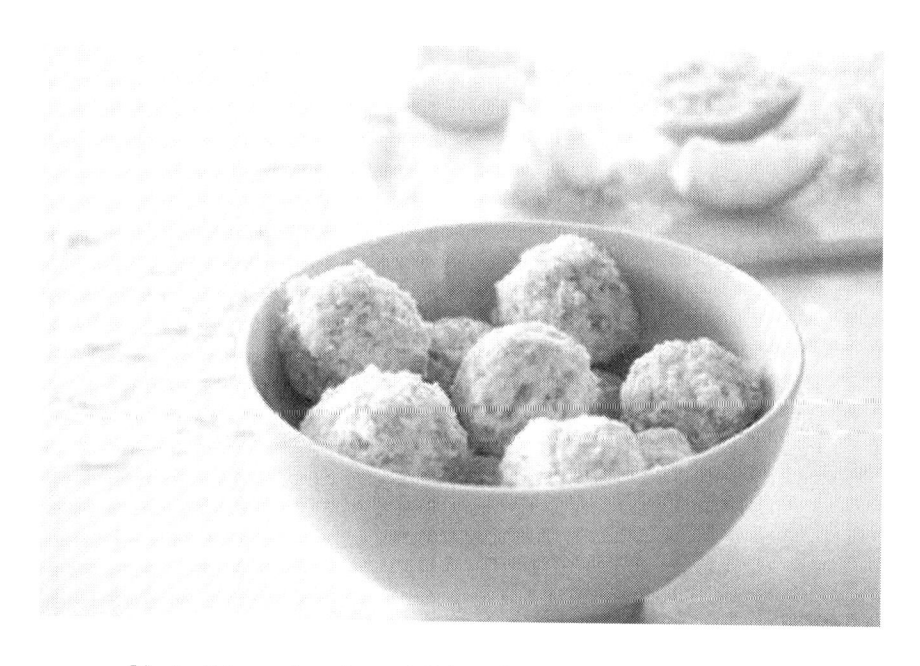

Nutritional value 131 cal
Protein 1.8 g
Fat 5 g
Carbohydrates 0.5 g

*An easy to prepare, healthy to eat, and amazingly addicting dessert recipe, keto macaroon fat bombs makes a perfect dessert idea if you were ever to throw a treat to a crowd!*

Serves: 10
Preparation time: 5 minutes
Cooking time: 8 minutes

## Ingredients

¼ cup almond flour, organic
½ cup shredded coconut
2 tbsp. swerve
1 tbsp. vanilla extract
1 tbsp. coconut oil
3 egg whites

## Instructions

1. In a medium bowl, add shredded coconut, almond flour, and swerve. Mix until well blended.
2. In a small saucepan, melt the coconut oil and add the vanilla extract to it.
3. Meanwhile, refrigerate a medium bowl for mounting the egg whites.
4. Add the four mixes to the melted coconut oil and blend really well.
5. Next, add the egg whites to the chilled bowl and whisk until stiff.
6. Slowly and gently add the egg whites into the flour mix, making sure it doesn't overmix.
7. Finely spoon the mixture into muffin cups.
8. Bake at 400 degree F until macaroons start to brown, for 8 minutes.
9. Remove from oven and allow them to cool before serving.

## Lunch Recipe 25 (Dessert)

# QUICK 3-INGREDIENTS PEANUT BUTTER FUDGE

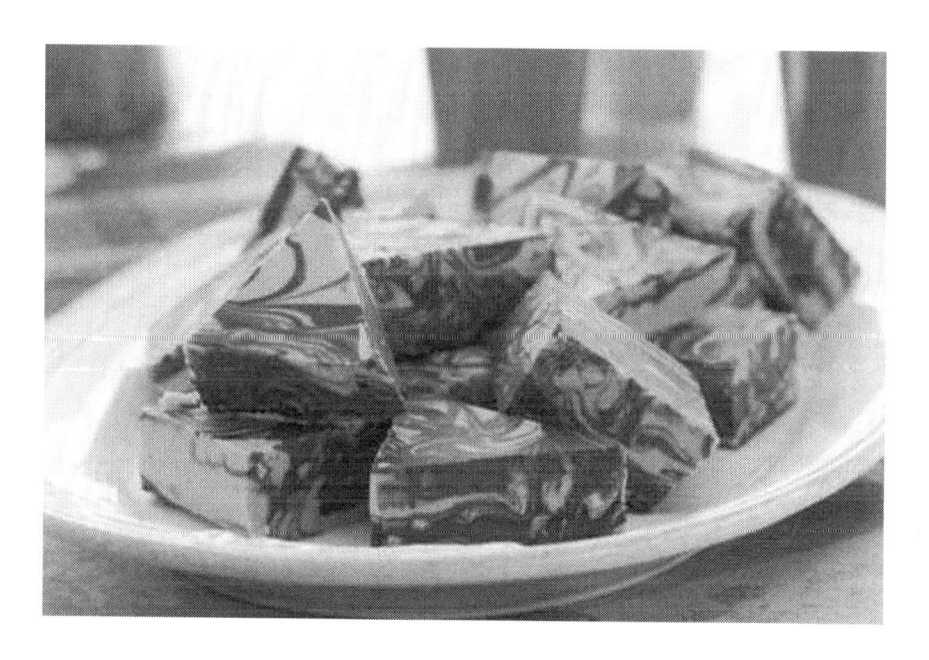

Nutritional value 287 cal
Protein 5 g
Fat 29 g
Carbohydrates 4 g

*What makes this marvellously elaborate dessert recipe a pure treat is its ketogenic nature. Get ready with your microwaves, as this good afternoon recipe is not only easy to prepare and amazing to eat, but also makes a perfect after-lunch dessert if you were ever to throw a treat to a crowd!*

Serves: 2
Preparation time: 5 minutes
Cooking time: 10 minutes

# Ingredients

1 cup peanut butter, unsweetened
1 cup coconut oil
¼ cup vanilla almond milk, unsweetened
2 tsp. desired sweetener, preferably stevia (optional)

### *Optional Topping: Chocolate Sauce*

¼ cup cocoa powder, unsweetened
2 tbsp. melted coconut oil
2 tbsp. Sweetener of choice

# Instructions

1. In a microwave or low-heat stove, melt the peanut butter and coconut oil slightly.
2. Add this melted mixture to your blender along with the rest of the ingredients and blend until well combined.
3. Add the mixture into a parchment lined loaf pan.
4. Freeze for about 2 hours.
5. If opted for chocolate sauce, whisk the ingredients first and then the sauce over fudge.
6. It's best to enjoy it after kept refrigerated overnight.

## Lunch Recipe 26 (Dessert)

## LOW CARB ALMOND FLOUR WAFFLES

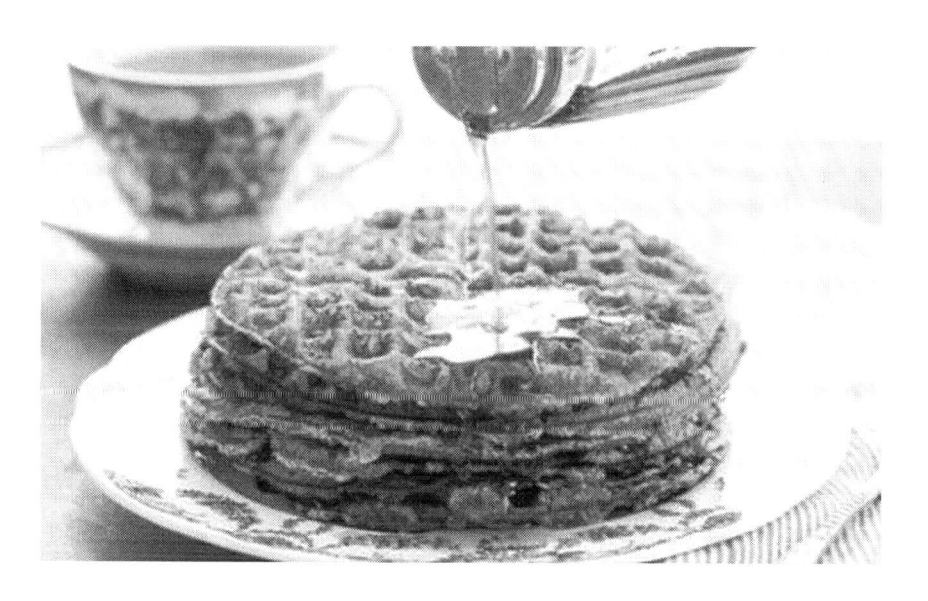

Nutritional value 237 cal
Protein 5 g
Fat 23 g
Carbohydrates 4 g

*An easy to prepare, healthy to eat, and amazingly addicting dessert recipe, keto almond flour waffles make a perfect dessert idea if you were ever to throw a treat to a crowd!*

Serves: 8
Preparation Time: 5 MINUTES
Cooking Time: 5 MINUTES

## Ingredients

- 1 cup sifted almond flour
- ½ tbsp. baking powder
- ¼ tsp. salt for taste
- ¼ tsp. xanthan gum (optional)
- 1 cup heavy cream
- 2 tbsp. oil
- 3 eggs

## Instructions

1. In large bowl, whisk together baking powder, almond flour, xanthan gum and salt.
2. Stir in eggs and oil. Mix until well blended.
3. **Note: The complete 1 cup of liquid is not used usually.** Slowly and gradually, add heavy cream until the desired thickness is reached. In case, your batter gets too thin, add in more almond flour to make it thicker.
4. Pour the batter into waffle maker and cook until desired crispiness is achieved. (5-10 minutes)

## Lunch Recipe 27 (Dessert)

## KETO CREAM CHEESE TRUFFLES

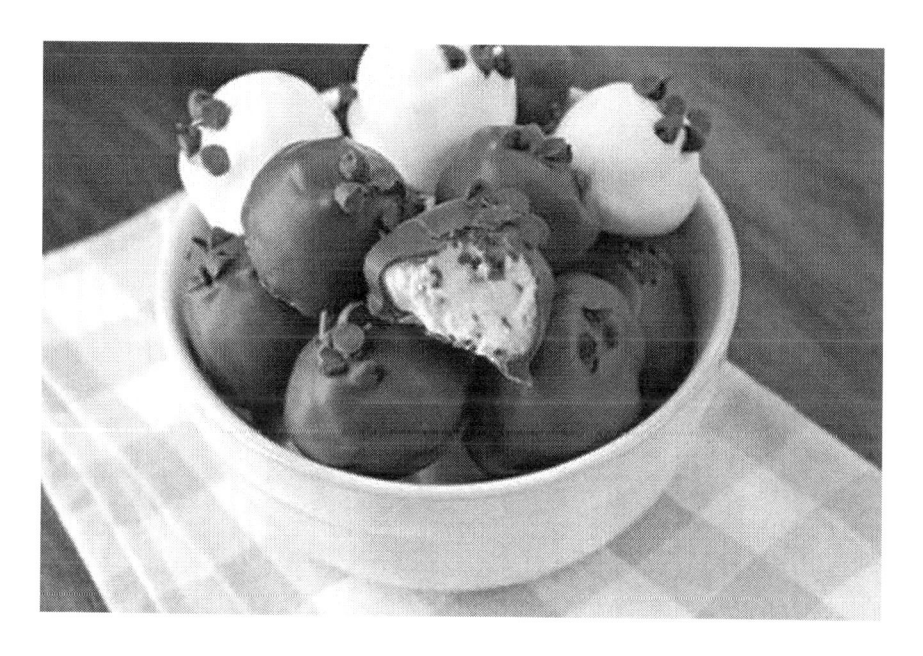

Nutritional value 72 cal
Protein 1.23 g
Fat 6 g
Carbohydrates 1.67 g

*Embrace yourself! This good afternoon dessert recipe is not only easy to prepare and amazing to eat, but also makes a perfect after-lunch dessert if you were ever to throw a treat to a crowd!*

Serves: 24
Preparation time: 10 minutes
Cooking time: 0 minutes

## Ingredients

16 ounces softened cream cheese
½ cup cocoa powder, unsweetened and divided
4 tbsp. swerve confectioners
¼ tsp. liquid Stevia
½ tsp. rum extract
1 tbsp. instant coffee
2 tbsp. water
1 tbsp. heavy whipping cream
Paper candy cups for serving

## Instructions

1. In a large bowl, add ¼ cup cocoa powder, cream cheese, stevia, swerve, rum extract, water, instant coffee, and heavy whipping cream.
2. Whip all the ingredients using an electric hand mixer until they are well combined. Refrigerate the bowl for half an hour to chill before rolling.
3. Next, spread out the left over cocoa powder. Roll the heaping tablespoons using the palms of your hands to form balls, and then roll them around in the cocoa powder. You should end up with around 20-24 balls in total. Place them in the small paper candy cups.
4. Refrigerate for an hour before serving.

## Lunch Recipe 28

## AVOCADO EGG SALAD

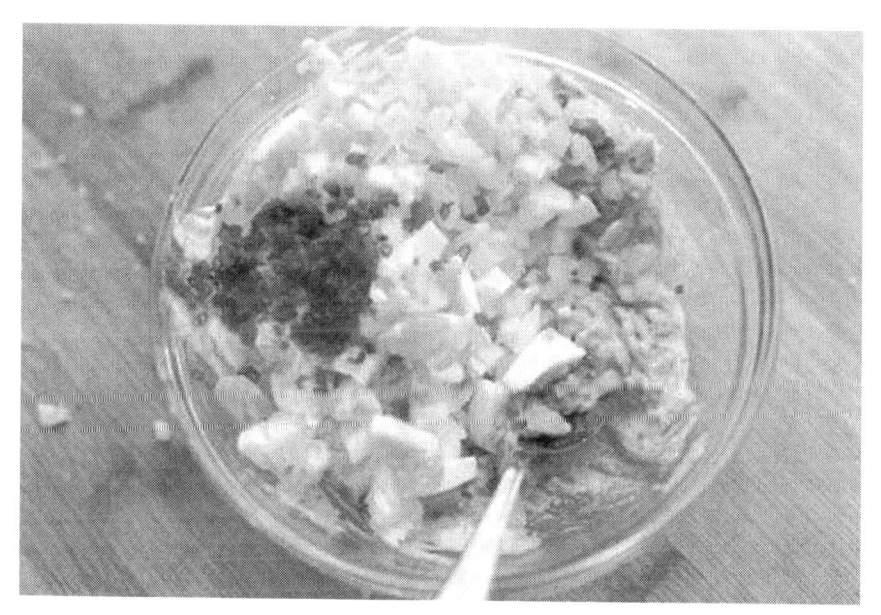

Image source: Inspired Taste

Nutritional value 155 cal
Protein 9 g
Fat 12 g
Carbohydrates 4.5 g

*An easy to prepare, healthy to eat, and amazingly addicting avocado keto egg salad is simply a perfect lunch idea if you were ever to throw a treat to a crowd! This recipe is perfectly Soy-free, Mayo-free, Whole 30 friendly and perfectly keto.*

Serves: 4
Preparation time: 5 minutes
Cooking time: 5 minutes

## Ingredients

5 peeled and boiled eggs
1 ripe avocado
4 slices bacon (sugar-free and nitrate-free) cooked till crumbled and crisp
2-3 finely sliced green onion
1½ tbsp freshly squeezed lemon juice
½ tsp sea salt, finely grained
Smoked paprika
Veggies to serve the dish with

## Instructions

1. Chop the boiled eggs and shift them to a large bowl.
2. Cut apart the avocado and remove the pit.
3. Add the ripe avocado into the bowl.
4. Next, Mash the avocado and combine well with the freshly chopped eggs.
5. Now, add salt and the lemon juice while mixing well.
6. Add the chives, crumbled bacon and sprinkle them with the smoked paprika.
7. Serve with an extra squeeze of lemon and fresh veggies. Enjoy!

*The amazing blend of avocados and eggs in a salad not only offers an absolute delight but also adds an extra-healthy parameter to this salad. So, this keto salad makes a perfect lunch this season.*

# Lunch Recipe 29

## BASIL SCRAMBLE

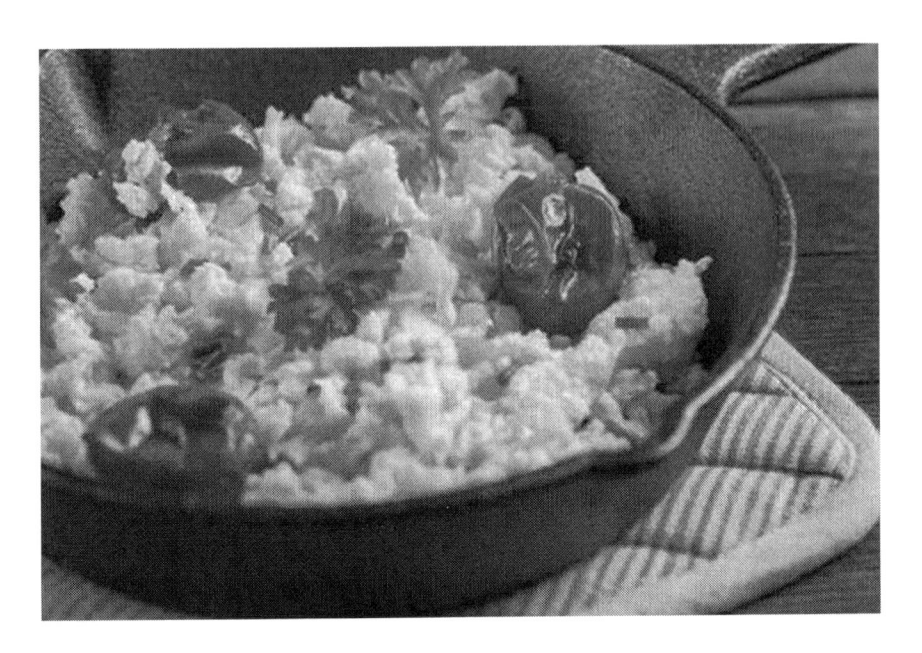

Nutritional value 205 cal
Protein 26 g
Fat 5 g
Carbohydrates 14 g

*A delicious lunch that is sure to become a prominent meal in your everyday life, the 'Gluten-free tomato basil scramble' incorporates the freshness of tomato and basil.*

Serves: 4
Preparation time: 5 minutes
Cooking time: 15 minutes

## Ingredients

- 4 sweet potatoes
- 1 tsp olive oil (extra-virgin)
- 1/3 cup water
- ¼ tsp kosher salt, for taste
- 4 tsp chives, finely chopped

## Instructions

1. Use a fork to prick sweet potatoes and rub them with oil.
2. Add potatoes and one-quarter cup of water in a baking dish (microwave-safe); and cover with a plastic wrap.
3. Now, Microwave at high until it gets tender, for at least 15 minutes, while regularly checking for its doneness every 5 minutes. Let it cool slightly.
4. Split the potatoes partially in half lengthwise; use a fork to fluff the flesh.
5. Drizzle with salt and top thoroughly with chives.

*The Keto tomato basil scramble recipe simply turns simple scrambled eggs into a marvelous treat. It ensures you a full and satisfied meal, no matter what. Enjoy!*

# Lunch Recipe 30

## POMEGRANATE CURRY CHICKEN

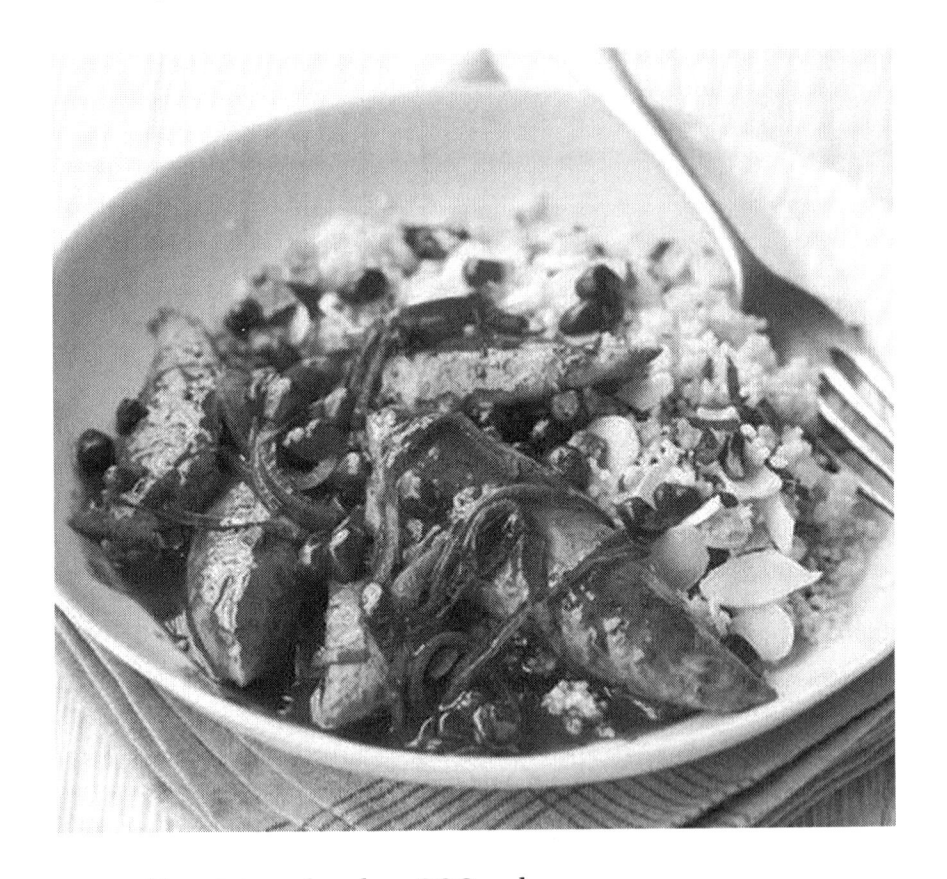

Nutritional value 238 cal
Protein 29 g
Fat 11 g
Carbohydrates 3 g

*No matter if you serve this easy and elegant pomegranate curry chicken with a bed of greens or with a side of steamed broccoli, it will quickly become your favorite recipe for lunch.*

Serves: 4
Preparation time: 10 minutes
Cooking time: 10 minutes

## Ingredients

3-oz. of boneless, skinless chicken thighs
1 tsp curry powder
½ tsp kosher salt
½ tsp black pepper for taste
1½ tsp olive oil (extra-virgin)
¼ cup pomegranate arils
2 tsp mint leaves, torn

## Instructions

1. Drizzle the whole of the chicken with salt, pepper and curry powder.
2. Pre-heat the oil over medium to high heat in a large-size skillet.
3. Add the chicken to this skillet and cook for the next 5 minutes on both the sides or until completely done.
4. Next, shift the chicken to the serving-platter.
5. You are ready to serve the chicken, just drizzle it with mint and pomegranate arils and enjoy a quick meal.

**This chicken dish makes a perfect lunch, as it requires handful of preparation and is ready to serve almost immediately. So get set for this dreamy lunch and enjoy!**

# Lunch Recipe 31

## BLACKENED STEAK SALAD

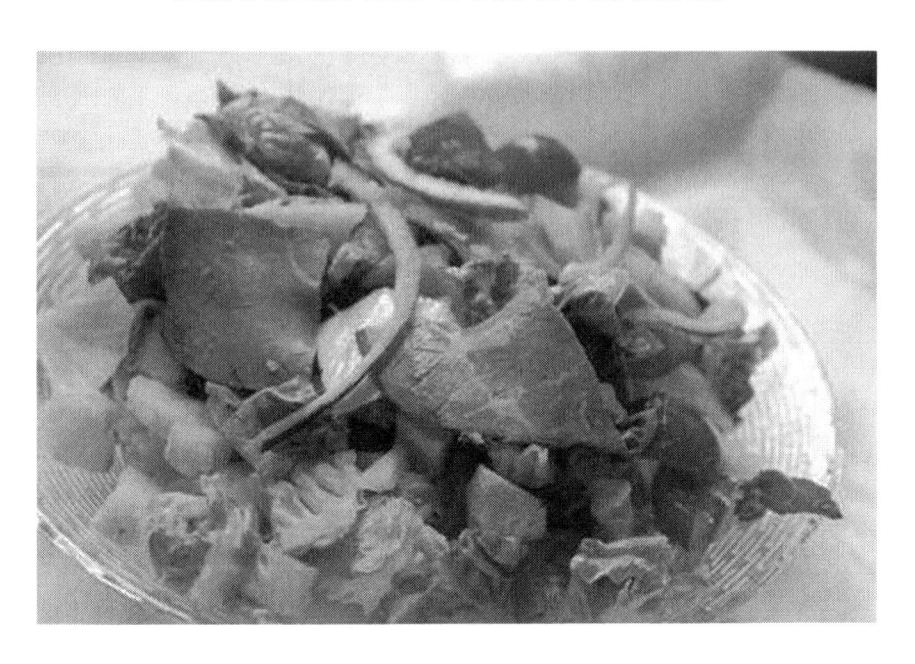

Nutritional value 332 cal
Protein 21 g
Fat 24.4 g
Carbohydrates 6 g

*Steak-centric salads often feature in the English gastro pub menu. Catering the royal menu to your doorsteps: this salad incorporates char grilled steak, topped with avocado and vinaigrette that elevates the veggies rather than disguise them. This recipe is not only healthy but also keto-friendly.*

Serves: 4
Preparation time: 15 minutes
Cooking time: 10 minutes

## Ingredients

½ tsp kosher salt
½ tsp black pepper
½ tsp paprika
¼ tsp garlic powder
12 oz. of trimmed flank steak
¼ cups of olive oil (extra-virgin)
2 tbsp balsamic vinegar
1 tsp Dijon mustard
4 cups arugula, firmly packed
½ red onion, vertically sliced
½ chopped ripe avocado

## Instructions

1. Take a grill pan and heat it over the medium to high heat.
2. In a small bowl add salt, pepper and garlic powder; mix it all thoroughly.
3. Rub the spice mixture thoroughly and evenly over the steak. Bring the steak into pan; let it grill for at least 5 minutes on both the sides until you reach the desired degree of doneness.
4. Keep the steak on to a cutting board. Let it cool for 5 minutes. Now, cut the grain into thin slices.

5. Next, mix vinegar, oil and mustard in a large bowl, while regularly stirring with a whisk.
6. Add arugula, steak and onion; toss to coat.
7. Divide salad among 4 plates and dress evenly with avocado.

**This is a Quick and Easy to prepare lunch salad recipe that is so very convenient, enriched with flavor, and tastes incredibly great. Enriched with the deliciousness, this lunch salad is relatively quick to be served as a lunch.**

## Lunch Recipe 32

## BUTTER SCALLOPS

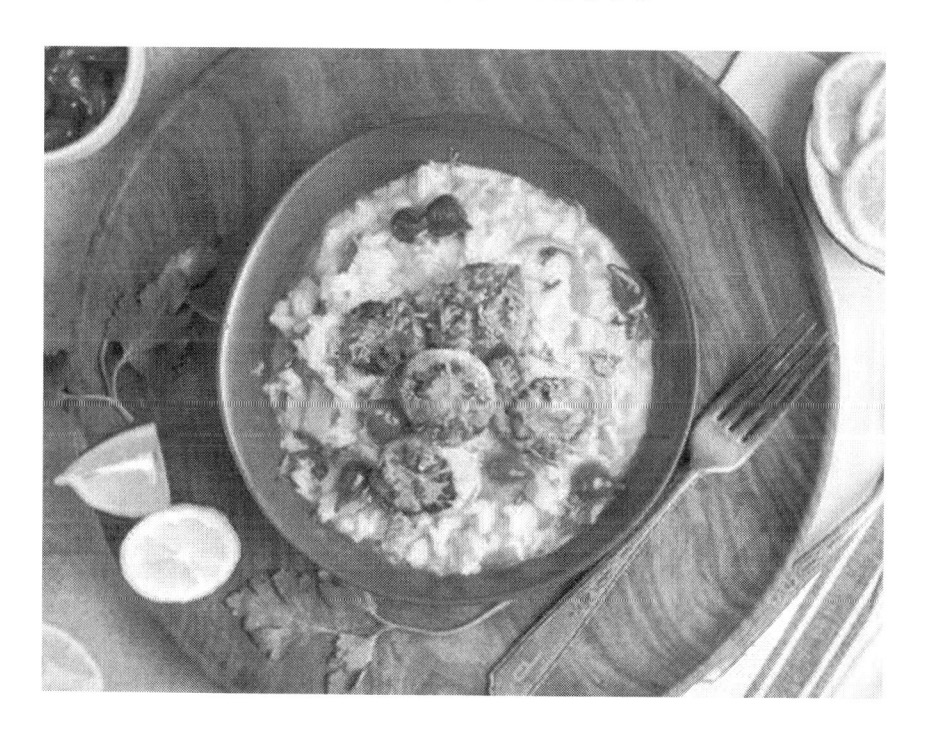

Nutritional value 215.6 cal
Protein 38.7 g
Fat 13.8 g
Carbohydrates 11.0 g

*If you are fond of the butter chicken, then you can get the same sort of taste only with these Keto Butter Scallops recipe. All it takes is one pan to combine everything as instructed in the tutorial and you are ready with your lunch within 25 minutes.*

Serves: 3-4
Preparation time: 10 minutes
Cooking time: 15 minutes

## Ingredients

2 tbsp ghee
1 cup of the minced shallot
2 tsp garlic paste (fresh)
2 tsp of fresh ginger paste
¼ cup of fresh tomato paste
½ tsp of salt for taste
1 tsp garam masala
Pinch of cayenne pepper
¼ tsp of ground cumin
¼ tsp of ground cinnamon
½ pound of sea scallops
8 ounces of cream' fraiche
Fresh cilantro for garnishing purpose

## Instructions

1. Heat the ghee over medium-high heat in a large skillet or wok pan.
2. Introduce the shallot and cook, while stirring gently and frequently, till the ingredient starts to get tender.
3. Bring in the ginger paste, garlic paste, tomato paste, garam masala, salt, cayenne, cumin, and cinnamon, and proceed towards cooking for the next 5 minutes.

4. Add the scallops and creme fraiche, continue cooking until the scallops are thoroughly cooked through.
5. Garnish with the fresh cilantro and serve.

*Ready to serve within 25 minutes from the start, the dish will cherish your name amongst your guests or it works wonders as just as a treat to yourself. And, last but not the least, it is Keto-approved.*

## Lunch Recipe 33

## SALMON SALAD

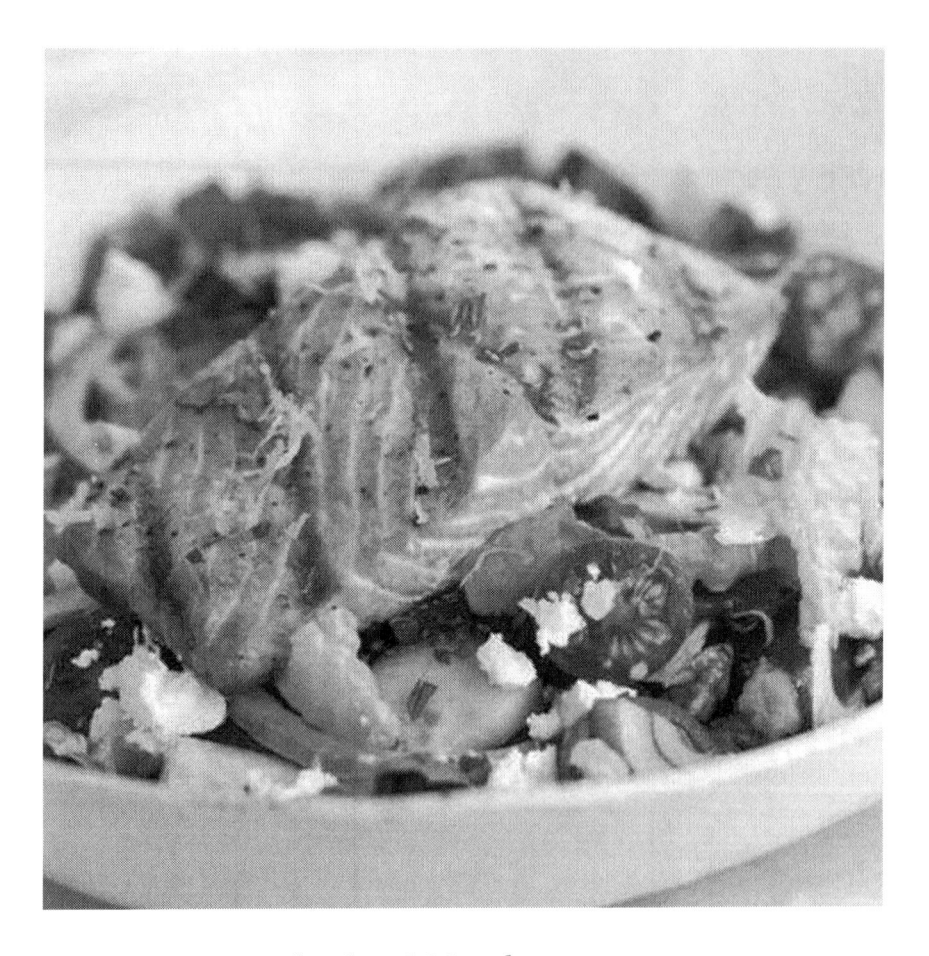

Nutritional value 200 cal
Protein 11 g
Fat 20 g
Carbohydrates 1 g

*This is one such insanely easily made dish, perfect for lunch on the go and also rich in protein and a good source of omega-3 fatty acids. Salmon Salad is a 5 minute cook.*

>Serves: 4
>Preparation time: 5 minutes
>Cooking time: 5 minutes

## Ingredients

>10-12 oz. canned mayonnaise
>4 tbsp celery chopped
>2 tbsp of chopped onion
>1/2 tsp. Dried dill
>A pinch of black pepper

## Instructions

1. Take a bowl and add the all the ingredients and toss them properly.
2. Take a kale leaf or collard, on a bed of greens, add veggies such as cucumber, tomato on the top and roll over.

*Life is busy, but don't let that disrupt your lifestyle in any way, choose this healthy option!*

## Lunch Recipe 34

## TOMATO AND BASIL CHICKEN

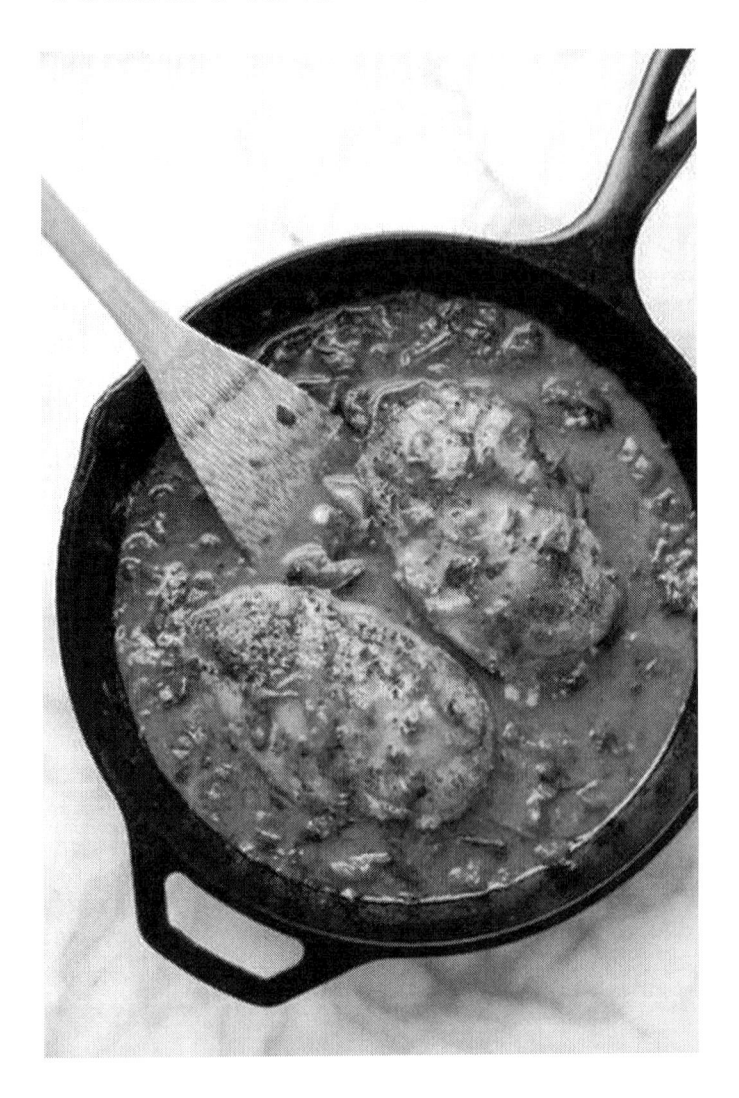

Nutritional value 220 cal
Protein 30 g
Fat 10 g
Carbohydrates 4 g

*Keto diets focus on grass-fed meats a lot, chicken is a great option for lunch. Give a tangy hint to your chicken, how about chicken tossed in pesto!*

Serves: 2
Preparation time: 10 minutes
Cooking time: 30 minutes

## Ingredients

2 pound chicken thighs/breasts, boneless and skinless
1 onion, yellow
2 teaspoon coconut oil
1 teaspoon arrowroot powder
½ cup cold water
1 cup coconut milk

**Nut-Free Dairy-Free Pesto:**

5 cloves of garlic
4 tbsp. sunflower seeds
2 ½ tbsp. nutritional yeast
Handful of salt & pepper
1 (2-3) oz. package fresh basil
2 tbsp. avocado oil

## Instructions

1. In a medium-sized skillet, heat coconut oil over medium-high or until it starts to sizzle.
2. Meanwhile, chop the onion into strips; add to the pan; cook until it becomes translucent.

3. Next, add chicken; cook for another 15 minutes; flip over; cook for 15 more minutes or until there's no pink in the middle of the chicken.

**Prepare the pesto:**

1. Add garlic in a food processor; Pulse until finely minced. Next, add sunflower seeds, pulse.
2. Add nutrition yeast, salt, and a dash of pepper to the food processor. Lastly, add avocado oil and basil.
3. Pulse until the basil is well minced. Meanwhile, as you prepare the recipe, you could set the pesto aside.
4. In a bowl, add arrowroot powder and water and whisk them together.
5. Add the coconut milk, and then whisk in the pesto.
6. Add the sauce to the chicken resting within the skillet and bring it to simmer.
7. Add the sliced cherry tomatoes and let it simmer for another couple of minutes or until tomatoes become warm. Serve.

*This cuisine is a creamy yet tangy, you can serve this with zoodles as an optional method but it Serves: quite a meal itself*

# Lunch Recipe 35

## TUNA AND TOMATO BURGERS

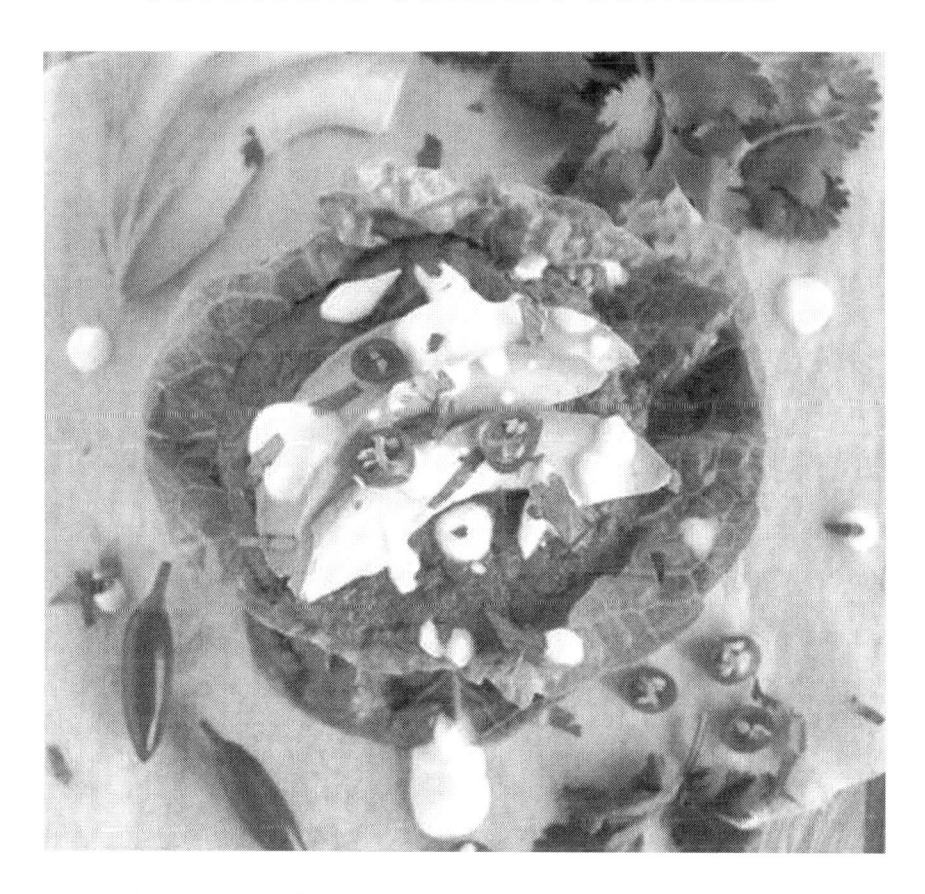

Nutritional value 150 cal
Protein 18 g
Fat 7 g
Carbohydrates 4 g

**Burgers for lunch? Yes! Burgers for lunch!**

**Being keto should never stop you from being interesting and trying out various forms of other**

*dishes, such as this amazing burger, learn how to make this!*

## Ingredients

2 cup of tuna, drained and rinsed
2 red onion, finely chopped
2 red chili, finely chopped
1 crushed garlic clove
2 eggs
4 tbsp of tomato paste
1 tbsp of coconut flour
Salt and pepper to taste

### *For Serving*

Burger buns
Lettuce
Avocado
Extra chilli
Fresh coriander (cilantro)
Greek yoghurt

## Instructions

1. Heat your oven in advance at 1750 C (3500 F).
2. Line a baking sheet parchment paper and set aside.
3. Keep your burger's ingredients into a medium-large sized bowl and stir well till they are nicely combined.

4. Carefully roll and flatten the tuna mixture using your hands into 6, even sized burger Pattie. Finally place them on your baking tray.
5. Add in the microwave and cook for the next 10 minutes.
6. Serve immediately.

***This meal might not be as low carb as keto diets focus on but certainly is the best way to have as cheat meals without cheating whole with the keto routine!***

# Lunch Recipe 36

## BANANA NUT PORRIDGE

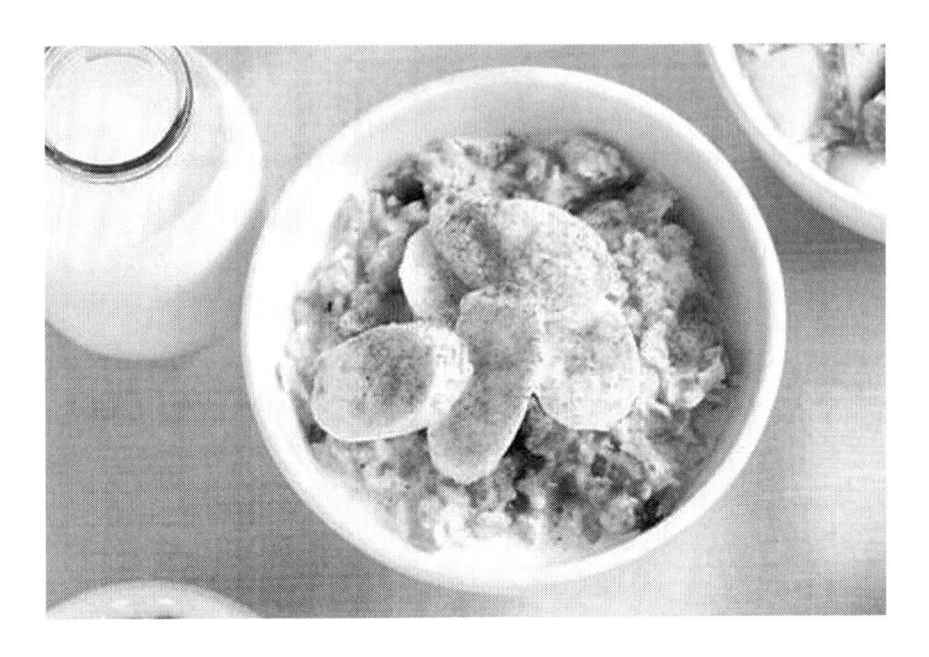

Nutritional value 239 cal
Protein 8 g
Fat 27 g
Carbohydrates 7 g

*Porridge is one amongst that ultimate form of lunch, after oats. Give it a banana spin to your normal porridge making it healthier and team it with nuts!*

## Ingredients

¼ cup cashews, raw
¼ cup almonds, raw

¼ cup pecans, raw
1 ripe banana
1 cup of coconut milk
1 tsp cinnamon
Dash of sea salt to soak water

## Instructions

1. Add the nuts in a large-sized bowl and drizzle the sea salt over them. Fill up the bowl with the filtered water to make sure that the nuts are covered by minimum 1 inch of water. Cover it thoroughly and soak throughout the night.
2. Drain off the nuts and wash for 2 or 3 times, till the water runs clear.
3. Bring the drained nuts within a high speed blender or a food processor. Mix the nuts together with the coconut milk, banana, and cinnamon until the mixture becomes smooth.
4. Distribute the ingredients among the bowl and let it microwave for nearly 40 seconds.
5. Serve with chopped nuts, raisins and an extra splash of milk if desired.

*Rich with nutrients and warm flavors, but unfortunately a little less liked by kids, add waffles with this porridge recipe to have the perfect lunch!*

## Lunch Recipe 37

## COCONUT CHICKEN FINGERS

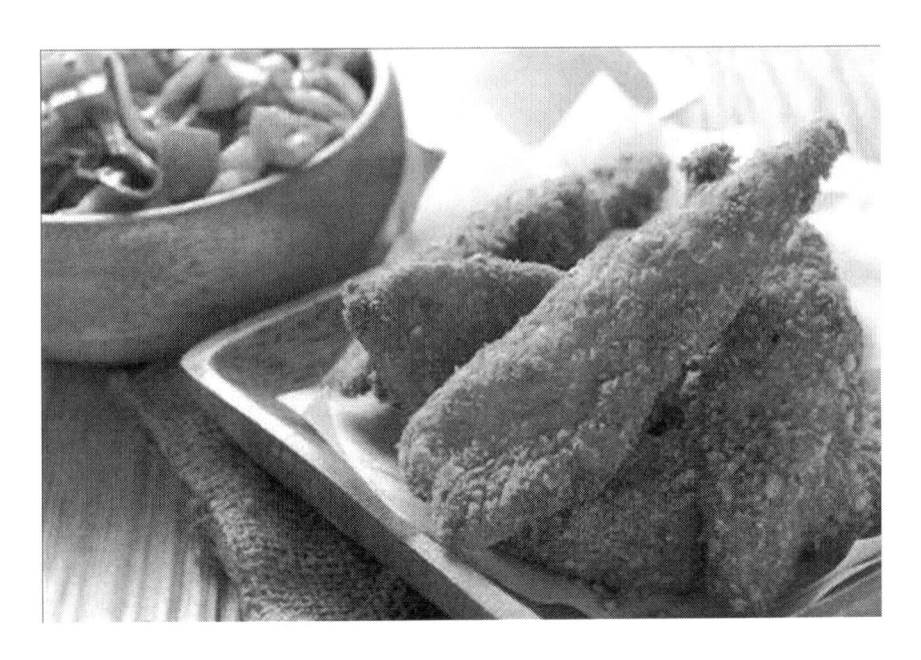

Nutritional value 298 cal
Protein 28 g
Fat 12 g
Carbohydrates 0 g

*Chicken tenders are Keto and Glutten free in nature and are easy and quick meal to make. We recommend you to double the recipe and heat them again and again throughout the entire week for extra fast lunchs.*

Serves: 4
Preparation time: 5 minutes
Cooking time: 20 minutes

## Ingredients

1 pound of skinless and boneless chicken tenders
1 egg
½ cup of cashew flour
1 cup coconut, unsweetened and shredded
¼ tsp salt for taste
¼ pepper for taste
¼ tsp garlic powder
¼ tsp cinnamon

## Instructions

1. Heat the oven in advance at 375 degrees.
2. Whisk the eggs in a large bowl and set them aside.
3. Mix coconut, cashew flour and spices in a different dish or a bowl.
4. Lightly dip each chicken tender/finger in the whisked egg followed by dipping in the batter
5. Take a baking sheet lined with a parchment paper and keep the coated chicken tenders on it.
6. Next, bake for at least 15 minutes or until the tenders get golden brown in color and there's no pink on the inside.

*The combination of chicken fingers and coconut makes a great lunch and sure to be your secret best friends. In fact the combination has a great potential to make you fall in love with it. The recipe is quite easy and convenient to prepare and doesn't require anything else to be a complete meal.*

## Lunch Recipe 38

## GLUTTEN-FREE EGG ROLL IN BOWL

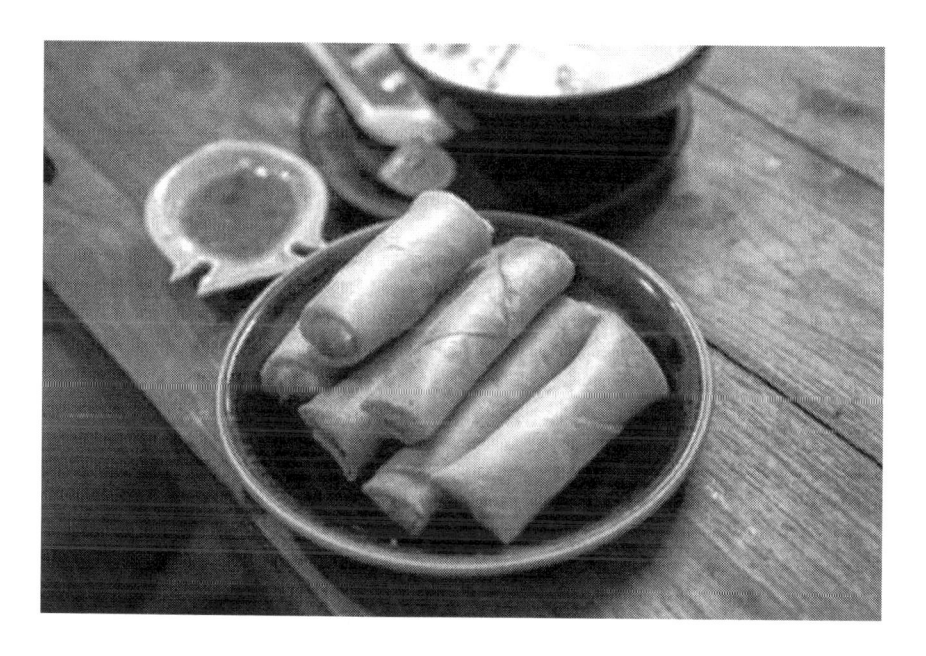

Nutritional value 200 cal
Protein 8 g
Fat 1.5 g
Carbohydrates 20 g

*This meal not only focuses on low carb diet, but is also the best way to have a delicious meal without compromising on your keto-diet routine. So, embrace yourself and start your afternoon with the egg roll in the bowl.*

Serves: 12
Preparation time: 15 minutes
Cooking time: 25 minutes

## Ingredients

1 small cabbage head finely chopped into slices
2 medium carrots, chipped into long strips
1 tbsp coconut oil, unflavoured
½ cup of coconut aminos
1 ½ tbsp of the sesame oil
2 minced garlic cloves
3 diced green onions

## Instructions

1. Melt the unflavoured coconut oil at medium to high heat.
2. Add cabbage and the carrot.
3. Sautee until the mixture gets soft. Or else if it becomes extra dry, then add water and allow it to evaporate and soften the mixture.
4. Next, add in the sesame oil and the coconut aminos.
5. Keep boiling until it gets softer and the sauce is thoroughly absorbed.
6. Now, bring in the garlic and keep cooking until it gets fragrant.
7. Add the green onions at the top of the mixture.

*This amazing keto egg roll in a bowl has earned itself the reputation of bringing huge smiles on faces, so no matter if you have to throw a house party to your loved ones or a little bash with your partner, this Keto recipe will never disappoint you.*

## Lunch Recipe 39

## QUICK AND EASY LUNCH SCRAMBLE

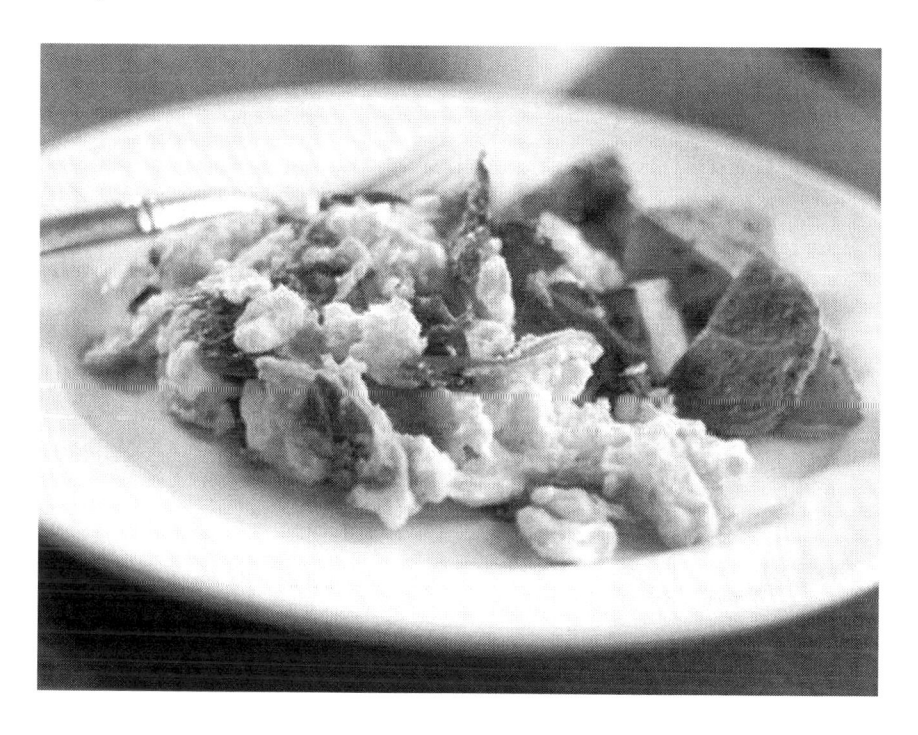

Nutritional value 199.3 cal
Protein 13 g
Fat 15 g
Carbohydrates 2 g

*What makes this marvellously elaborate recipe a pure treat is its gluten-free nature. Get ready with your muffin try, as this good morning recipe is not only easy to prepare and amazing to eat, but also makes a perfect lunch idea if you were ever to throw a treat to a crowd!*

Serves: 1
Preparation time: 10 minutes
Cooking time: 10 minutes

## Ingredients

3 whisked eggs
4 mushrooms (baby bella)
1/3 cup of the red- peppers
½ cup spinach
Deli ham, 2 slices
1 tbsp ghee or coconut oil
Salt and pepper to taste

## Instructions

1. Chop the vegetables and the ham together.
2. Keep ½ tbsp of butter into a frying pan and allow it to melt. Sauté the hams and vegetables together.
3. Take a separate frying pan and add the whisked eggs and ½ tbsp of butter.
4. Allow this mixture to be cooked on medium-high heat while stirring for in order to prevent overcooking.
5. When the eggs are cooked thoroughly, season them with pepper and salt accordingly.
6. Last but not the least, combine the saute'd vegetables and ham with the egg mix.
7. Serve immediately.

*Quick and easy, this lunch scramble is keto in nature and is easy and quick meal to make. We recommend you to double the delight of the recipe by sharing it with your loved ones as a great lunch.*

## Lunch Recipe 40

# GOOD NOON CHICKEN BURRITO BOWLS

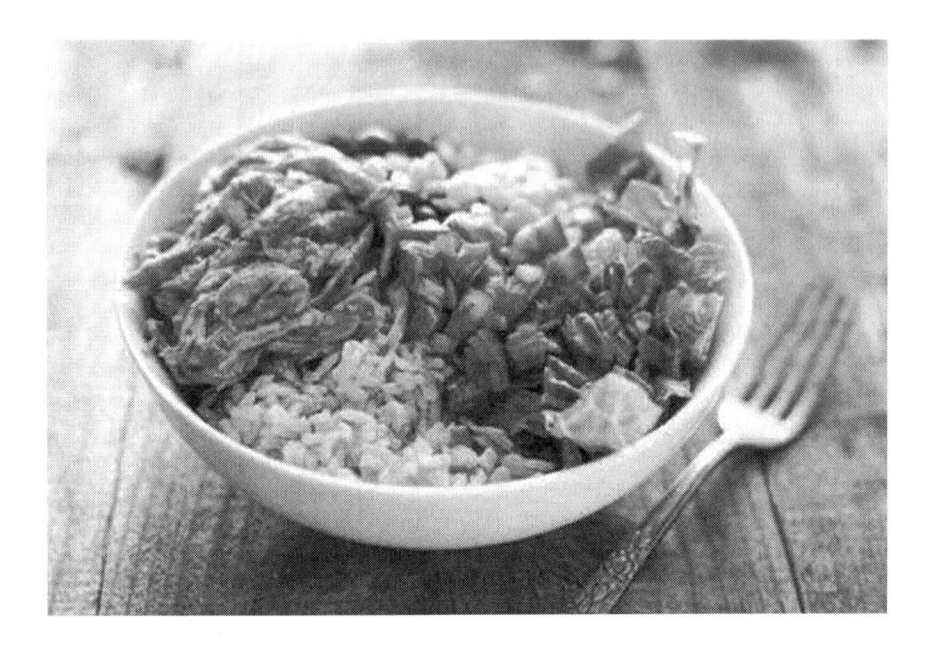

Nutritional value 350 cal
Protein 14 g
Fat 21 g
Carbohydrates 9 g

*This good noon chicken burrito bowls not only focuses on low carb diet, but also Serves: the pinnacle of delight to your taste buds. So, sit back and relax, your afternoon is all set to be enlightened by this burrito bowl.*

Serves: 4
Preparation time: 10 minutes
Cooking time: 20 minutes

## Ingredients

2 cups of kale
1 ½ cups of grape tomatoes
3 cups of cubed or shredded chicken
¾ cup of canned corn
2 cups of canned black beans
1 cup of cooked rice
1 ½ tsp paprika
½ tsp of cumin
1/3 tsp of cayenne
1/3 tsp pepper

## Instructions

1. Follow the directions to prepare rice or you could purchase the cooked rice as well.
2. Mix the rice in cumin, paprika, cayenne, and pepper and let them cook with rice for about 5 minutes.
3. Coat the container or the bowl to be used with tomatoes, kale, rice, corn and beans.
4. You are ready to serve.

***This amazing burrito bowl has long known for pleasing the crowd, so no matter if you have to throw a house party to your loved ones or a little bash with your partner, this Keto recipe will never disappoint you.***

## Lunch Recipe 41

## PIZZA FRITTATA

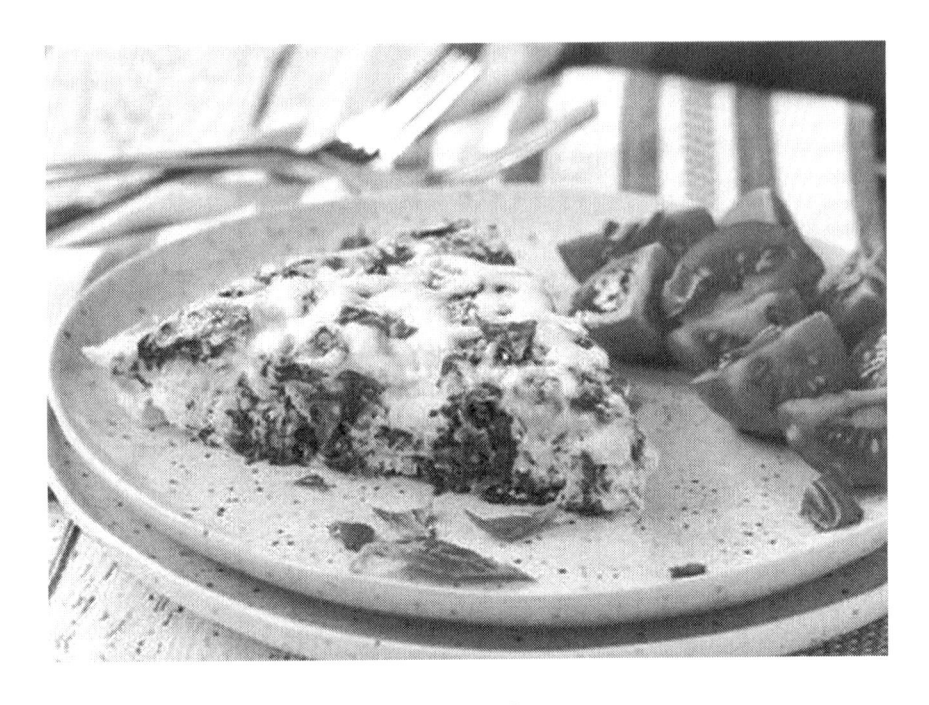

Nutritional value 314 cal
Protein 23 g
Fat 20 g
Carbohydrates 11 g

*If you think pizza cannot be healthy then you are yet to come across this magician dish called the keto pizza frittata. Served with the typical pizza sauce, it will soon take over the place of your favourite recipe.*

Serves: 10
Preparation time: 35 minutes
Cooking time: 8 minutes

## Ingredients

½ pound Italian sausage
6 eggs
1 cup of pizza sauce
1/3 cup of fresh basil, worn out into small pieces
Pinch of salt, pepper and red pepper for taste
½ sliced green bell pepper
4 sliced button mushrooms
4 slices of pepperoni
2 cups of arugula
Fresh lemon juice from ½ lemons

## Instructions

1. Heat the oven in advance at 350 degrees F.
2. Heat the skillet over medium-high heat.
3. Bring in the sausage while using a wooden spoon to divide it into smaller pieces, till there is no pink visible.
4. Deliberately layer the sausage across the skillet.
5. Turn down the heat to medium-low.
6. Take a large bowl; beat the eggs together with basil, salt, pepper, pizza sauce and red pepper flakes.

7. Add this mixture into skillet and allow it to cook in the pan for at least 5 minutes.
8. Dress the frittata using the mushrooms, green pepper slices, and pepperoni. Now, keep it in the oven and bake for 20 minutes.
9. Pitch arugula in olive oil and lemon and keep it on the top of frittata just before serving!

***Just when you were bored of the typical lunch recipes, this frittata paved its way to our recipe book and came to your health and taste bud's rescue. Enjoy a rich blend of taste and health with this amazing recipe and thank us later.***

## Lunch Recipe 42

## EGG MUFFIN RECIPE

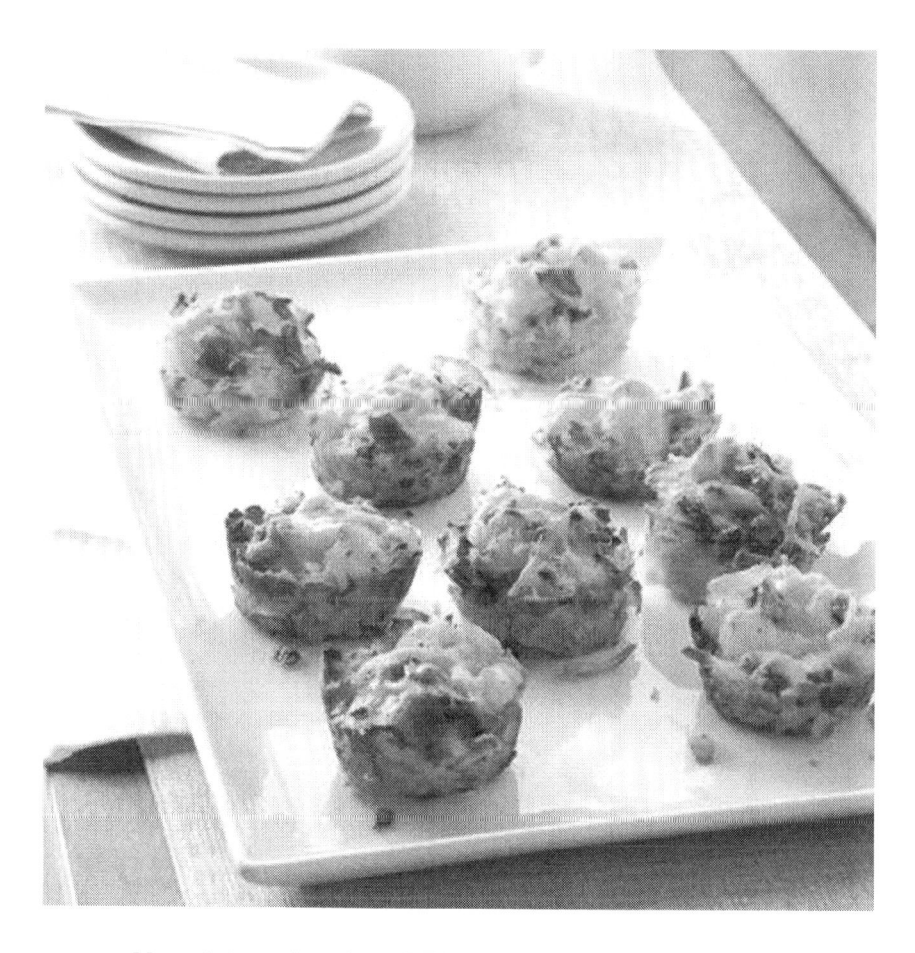

Nutritional value 250 cal
Protein 20.3 g
Fat 13 g
Carbohydrates 6.8 g

**This is a Quick and Easy to prepare Keto Egg muffin lunch recipe that is so very convenient, enriched**

with flavor, veggies and meat and tastes incredibly great. Jam packed with the deliciousness, these lunch muffins are relatively quick to be served as a lunch.*

Serves: 3
Preparation time: 5 minutes
Cooking time: 20 minutes

## Ingredients

6 eggs
8 ounces crumbled and cooked ham
1 ½ cup of red bell pepper, diced
1 cup onion, diced
¼ tsp salt, for taste
1 tsp. ground black pepper, for taste
2 tbsp. water

## Instructions

1. Preheat the oven to 170 degree C or 350 degrees F.
2. Drizzle 6 muffin cups and line them using a paper liner.
3. Take a large bowl and beat all the eggs within it.
4. Now, add ham, onion, bell pepper, salt, black pepper, and water into the beaten eggs.
5. Next, add the egg mixture evenly into each of the 6 muffin cups.

6. Bake the muffin cups in the preheated oven for at least 18 minutes until muffins find themselves set in the middle.

*This egg muffin lunch recipe is loaded with the goodness of a rich color, incorporated with healthy ingredient, thus making it a high protein and low carb meal.*

## Lunch Recipe 43

## EGG CASSEROLES

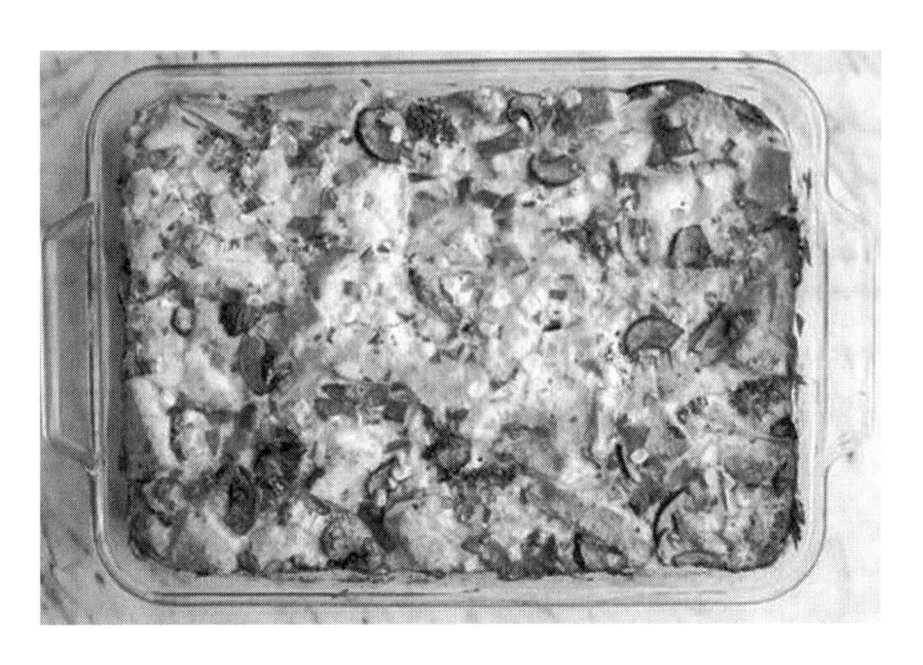

Nutritional value 334 cal
Protein 17 g
Fat 23 g
Carbohydrates 14 g

***An easy to prepare, healthy to eat, and amazingly addicting, Keto Egg Casseroles are simply a perfect lunch idea if you were ever to throw a treat to a crowd! This recipe is perfectly Soy-free, Mayo-free, Whole 30 friendly and perfectly keto.***

Serves: 4
Preparation time: 10 minutes
Cooking time: 10 minutes

## Ingredients

Keto Lunch Sausage, ½ lb
Diced Broccoli, ½ cup
½ diced Onion
6 Eggs
1 diced tomato
1 diced bell pepper
Sea Salt and black pepper to taste

## Instructions

1. Preheat the oven to 350 degrees F.
2. Add the eggs in a medium sized bowl and beat them until they start frothing.
3. Bring the onion, sausage, pepper, broccoli and tomato and stir well to combine these ingredients.
4. Distribute the mixture evenly among 6 different serving dishes.
5. Season with the sea salt and pepper.
6. Cook the mixture in the preheated oven for nearly 10 minutes, or till the eggs become firm.
7. Serve immediately.

## Lunch Recipe 44

### GRILLED FISH FILLET

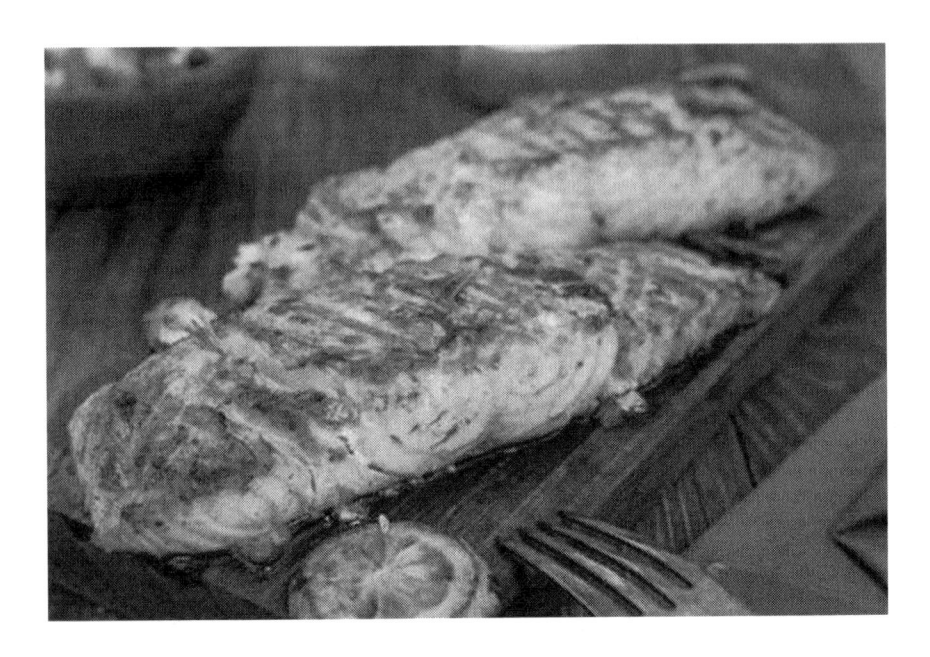

Nutritional value 123 cal
Protein 25.53 g
Fat 1.33 g
Carbohydrates 0.31 g

*This lunch couldn't have met a simpler fate. Made from the wholesome and delicious ingredients, these gluten-free grilled fish skillet is best served fresh, so prepare the skillet and gift yourself the luxury of a delicious fish skillet.*

Serves: 4
Preparation time: 10 minutes
Cooking time: 15 minutes

## Ingredients

- 4 (5 oz) of porgy fillets
- 4 teaspoons of olive oil
- Salt and freshly ground pepper, to taste
- 4 fresh sprig herbs (rosemary, parsley, oregano)
- 1 thinly sliced lemon
- 4 large pieces (20 inch) of heavy duty aluminum foil

## Instructions

1. Line the fish at the center of the foil.
2. Season with salt and pepper as per your taste while drizzling with olive oil.
3. Add a slice of lemon on the top of each fish piece, followed by a sprig of herbs on each.
4. Deliberately fold up the edges, to make sure that it's thoroughly sealed and no steam escaped.
5. Be careful in heating just one half of the grill on high heat while closing off the cover.
6. And when the grill is adequately hot, keep the foil packets beside the grill while the burner is turned off.
7. You can cook according to the thickness of your fish, for 10 to 15 minutes, or until it is adequately cooked through.

*The fusion of fillets and herbs is not only taste-full, but also takes this recipe to the pinnacle of deliciousness. So, the fish skillet makes a perfectly healthy treat this fall.*

## Lunch Recipe 45

## CILANTRO LIME SHRIMP WITH ZUCCHINI NOODLES

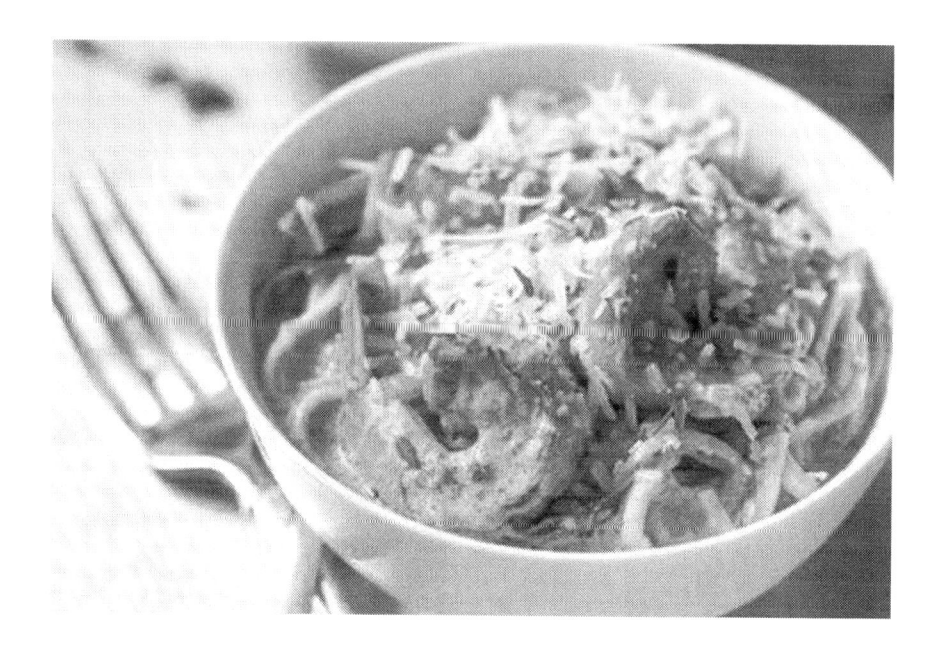

Serves: 4
Preparation time: 10 minutes
Cooking time: 15 minutes

*Just when you were bored of the typical lunch recipes, this zucchini pasta paved its way to our recipe book and came to your health and taste bud's rescue. Enjoy a rich blend of taste and health with this amazing recipe and thank us later.*

Nutritional value 347 cal
Protein 25.53 g
Fat 20 g

Carbohydrates 16 g

## Ingredients

2 tablespoons butter
1 pound of shelled jumbo shrimp
4 finely chopped garlic cloves
1 pinch red pepper flake
¼ cup white wine or chicken broth or shrimp broth or vegetable broth
2 tbsp lime juice
3 medium sized finely chopped noodle like zucchini
Salt and pepper to taste
1 tbsp lime zest
2 tbsp chopped cilantro

## Instructions

1. Over medium to high heat, melt the butter in a pan until it achieves frothing.
2. Add the shrimp followed by cooking for 2 minutes, flipping, bringing in the garlic and red pepper flakes(optional) and cook the ingredients for 1 more minute before keeping the shrimp aside.
3. Introduce the white wine and lime juice to the pan, deglaze it and boil the ingredients for the next 2 minutes.
4. Add the zucchini noodles and cook until they get delicate and supper, for about 2 minutes,

before dressing the ingredients with salt and pepper while adding the shrimp, lime zest and cilantro, tossing everything and removing from the heat.

## Lunch Recipe 46

## SAUTED CHICKEN MUSHROOM OMLETTE

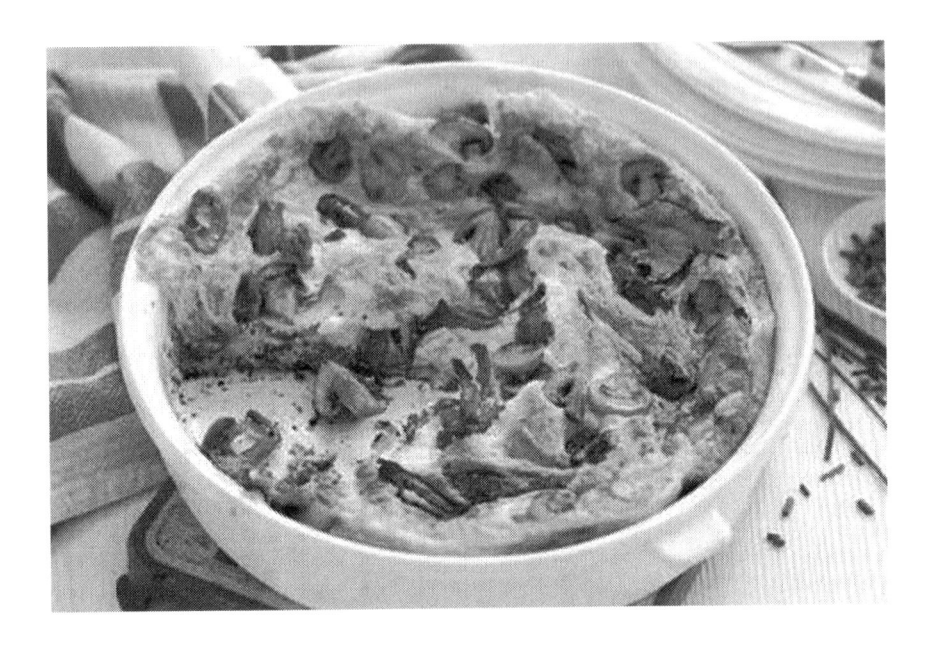

Serves: 4
Preparation time: 15 minutes
Cooking time: 5 minutes

*An easy to prepare, healthy to eat, and amazingly addicting, Chicken Mushroom Omlette is simply a perfect lunch idea if you were ever to throw a treat to a crowd! This recipe is perfectly Soy-free, Mayo-free, Whole 30 friendly and perfectly keto.*

Nutritional value 224 cal
Protein 18.5 g
Fat 14.8 g

Carbohydrates 4.1 g

## Ingredients

An egg along with 3 egg whites
1 tbsp parmesan cheese
1 tbsp cheddar cheese (shredded)
¼ tbsp sea salt (for taste)
1/3 tbsp red pepper flakes (crushed)
1/3 tbsp garlic powder
1/3 tbsp ground pepper
1/2 cup mushrooms (sliced)
2 tbsp green peppers (finely chopped)
1 tbsp onion (finely chopped)
1/2 tbsp olive oil
A cup of chicken sausage cut into slices

## Instructions

1. Beat the egg and egg whites in a small bowl.
2. Mix well the cheeses, salt, pepper flakes, garlic powder and pepper, and place it aside.
3. Sauté the mushrooms, green pepper and onions in an 8 inch non-sticky skillet for as many as 5 minutes or until it gets tender.
4. Add chicken sausage while continuing to cook and stir unless and until the chicken gets warm.
5. Introduce the egg mixture.
6. As the eggs take time to set in, you could lift edges while allowing the uncooked portion to smoothly flow underneath.

7. Chop into fine wedges in order to serve immediately.

## Lunch Recipe 47

## BAKED EGGS

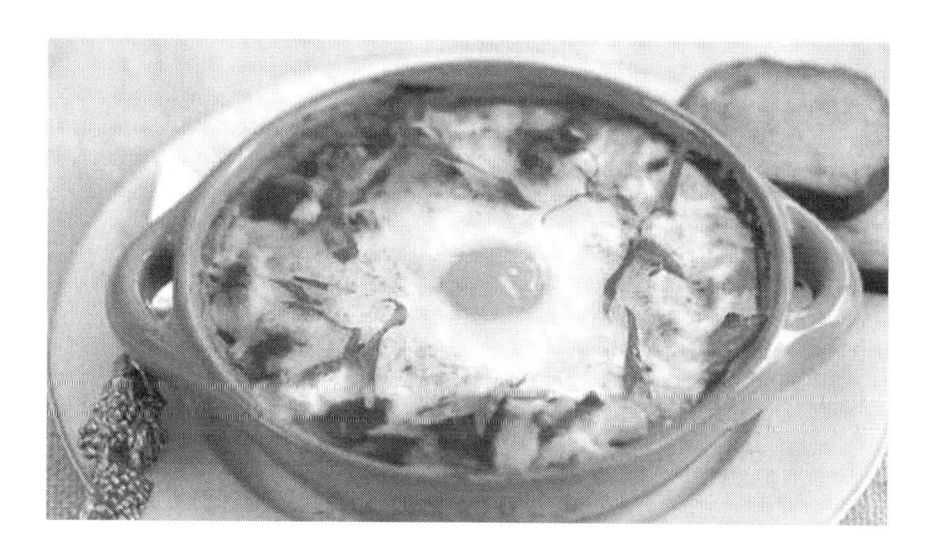

Serves: 6
Preparation time: 5 minutes
Cooking time: 30 minutes

*A delicious lunch that is sure to become a prominent meal in your everyday life, these 'Keto baked eggs' feature the freshness of raw eggs with the whipping cream.*

Nutritional value 143 cal
Protein 13 g
Fat 10 g
Carbohydrates 1 g

## Ingredients

1 tbsp. butter
6 eggs (medium to large)
1 tbsp. ground black pepper (fresh)
¾ tbsp. salt (for taste)
2 tbsp. cream (whipped)
6 ramekins or custard cups (6 ounce each)

## Instructions

1. Preheat the oven to 350° C.
2. Coat each of the 6 custard cups or the ramekins with ½ tbsp of butter.
3. Break an egg into each prepared custard cup or the ramekin.
4. Sprinkle the pepper and salt thoroughly over the eggs.
5. Combine each egg with the 1 tbsp of cream.
6. Keep each of the 6 ramekins or the custard cups in a baking dish (13x9 inch) and introduce the hot water within the pan till the height of 1 and ¼ inches.
7. Bake the mixture at 350° C for the next 30 minutes until the eggs are set.

> **TIP**
>
> Add Italian herbs to the baked eggs while serving and try with the lemon-pepper seasoning to add flavour to the recipe.

## Lunch Recipe 48

# CHICKEN THIGHS WITH SHALLOTS AND SPINACH

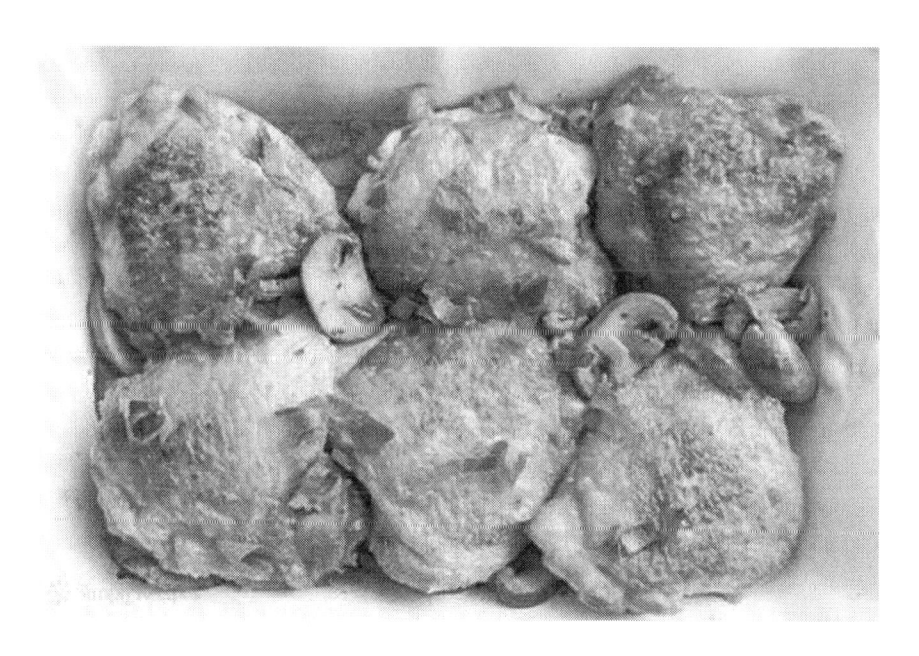

Nutritional value 224 cal
Protein 24 g
Fat 10 g
Carbohydrates 8 g

*Keto diets focus on grass-fed meats, and chicken is a great option for a low carb lunch. Give a tangy hint to your chicken, how about chicken shallots and spinach?*

Serves: 6
Preparation time: 10 minutes
Cooking time: 30 minutes

## Ingredients

6 boneless skinless chicken thighs (about 1-1/2 pounds)
1/2 teaspoon seasoned salt
1/2 teaspoon pepper
1-1/2 teaspoons olive oil
4 shallots, thinly sliced
1/3 cup white wine or reduced-sodium chicken broth
1 package (10 ounces) fresh spinach, trimmed
1/4 teaspoon salt
1/4 cup fat-free sour cream

## Instructions

1. Bring in the chicken and sprinkle it with seasoned salt and pepper.
2. Heat oil over medium to high heat, within a large non-sticky skillet finely coated with the cooking oil or the spray.
3. Mix in the chicken to the skillet while you cook it for the next 6 minutes on either sides or until the thermometer gives a reading of 170°.
4. Take the chicken away from the pan while ensuring that it remains warm yet fresh.
5. Cook and stir shallots in the same pan unless and until they become soft and tender. Then mix wine into the mixture and bring it to the boil.

6. Keep cooking till the wine decreases by half. Merge in the spinach and salt as per your requirements, as you cook and stir the ingredients until the spinach starts to wilt.
7. Stir in sour cream and serve with chicken, and you are ready to begin.

## Lunch Recipe 49

# SPINACH AND CHEDDAR MICROWAVE QUICHE

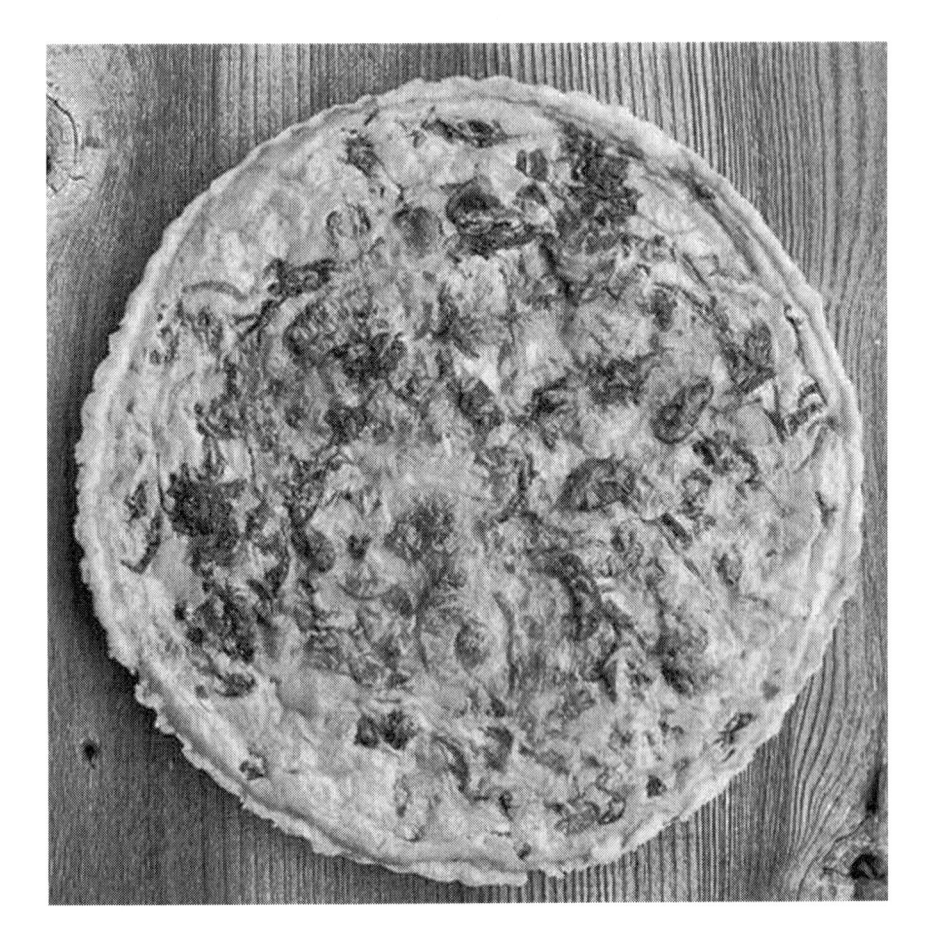

Serves: 1
Preparation time: 5 minutes
Cooking time: 3 minutes

*This meal not only focuses on low carb diet, but is also the best way to have a delicious meal without compromising on your keto-diet routine. So, embrace yourself and start your afternoon with this cheddar microwave quiche.*

Nutritional value 355 cal
Protein 11 g
Fat 29 g
Carbohydrates 20 g

## Ingredients

½ cup finely chopped spinach (frozen, thawed and properly drained)
1 egg
⅓ Cup of low fat milk
⅓ Cup of cheddar cheese (shredded)
1 chopped slice of bacon (cooked)
Salt and pepper just to taste

## Instructions

1. Keep the freshly chopped spinach in a mug incorporating couple of teaspoons of water. Cover the apparatus with a paper towel, while keeping the microwave on high temperature for almost one straight minute.
2. Take the apparatus off the microwave and drain the excess water or liquid from the spinach thoroughly.
3. Next, break the egg within the mug, adding it to the spinach and milk, complimented by cheese

and bacon. (Additionally add some salt and pepper as per your taste)
4. Mix the apparatus until and unless it combines perfectly well. Cover closely with a paper towel and microwave the apparatus on high temperature for 3 minutes.

## Lunch Recipe 50

# CHICKEN BREASTS WITH SHAVED BRUSSELS SPROUTS

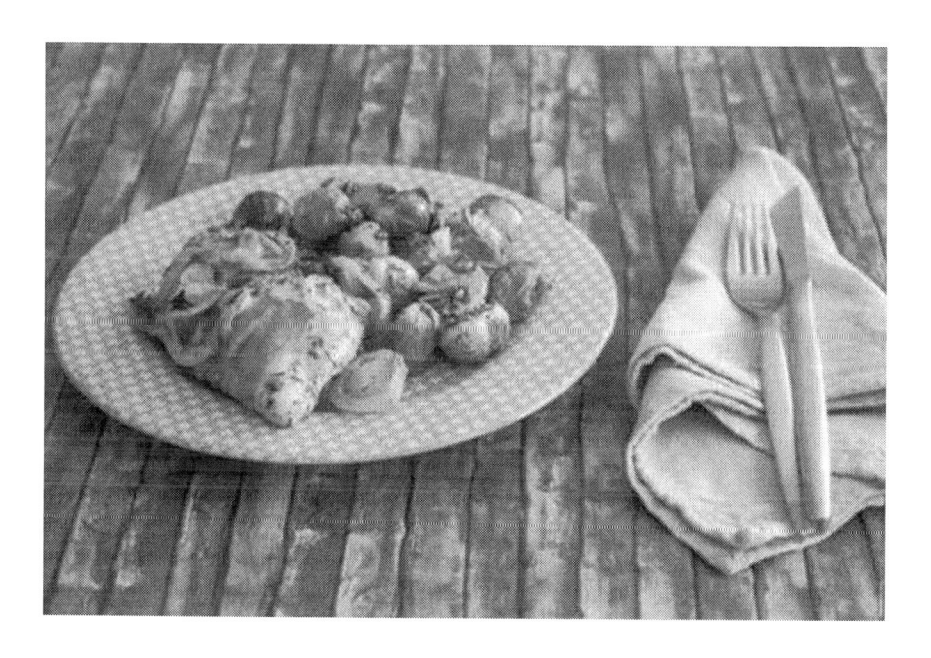

Nutritional value 355 cal
Protein 31 g
Fat 17 g
Carbohydrates 10 g

*The fusion of chicken breasts and Brussels sprouts is not only taste-full, but also takes this recipe to the pinnacle of deliciousness. This keto recipe makes a perfectly healthy treat this fall.*

Serves: 4
Preparation time: 10 minutes
Cooking time: 25 minutes

## Ingredients

2 (8-ounce) boneless, skinless chicken breast halves
3/4 teaspoon kosher salt, divided
2 broccoli stems
2 tbsp olive oil
2 tbsp fresh lemon juice
1/4 teaspoon freshly ground black pepper
3 cups thinly sliced Brussels sprouts (from 12 medium)
2 celery stalks, thinly sliced
¼ cup toasted hazelnuts
¼ cup fresh flat-leaf parsley, coarsely
Chopped 1 ounce Parmesan cheese, coarsely grated

## Instructions

1. In a small saucepan, keep the chicken and ½ teaspoon salt and cover with water; boiling the ingredients together. Instantly take them away from heat, get them covered, and let stand firm for the next 15 minutes.
2. Drain the chicken and let it stay under the cold water. As it cools completely; set it apart.
3. In the meantime, utilize a vegetable peeler to take away the outer layer of broccoli stems, focusing the major attention on the long strips.
4. Whisk together oil, quarter teaspoon salt and pepper, lemon juice in a large nonstick skillet,

5. Bring in broccoli strips, celery, hazelnuts, Brussels sprouts, parsley, and reserved chicken to bowl with dressing; and toss together to coat firmly.
6. Top the recipe with cheese.

Made in the USA
San Bernardino, CA
05 July 2018